Membership of the College Committee on Ethical Issues in Medicine

Sir Leslie Turnberg MD PRCP (*President*)
Sir Douglas Black MD FRCP Hon FFOM (*Convener*)
P Beck MD FRCP
J F L Aldridge OBE FRCP FFOM
S R Bloom MD DSc FRCP
M Bobrow CBE FRCP FRCPath
* The Reverend Professor G R Dunstan CBE DD LLD Hon FRCP
D C Evered MD FRCP
G R Ford CB FRCP
E Z R Gillon FRCP
J Grimley Evans MD FRCP
* Andrew Grubb MA
J S Horner FFPHM
* The Rt Hon Baroness Jay of Paddington
D N S Kerr CBE MB FRCP
D R London DM FRCP
* Sue MacGregor OBE Hon MRCP
M D Rawlins MD FRCP
M R Sanderson MRCP(UK)
J Saunders MD FRCP
* I Singh JP
J D Swales MD FRCP
J H Tripp MD FRCP
N J Wald FRCP

Observer
E Gadd MBChB MRCPsych (*Department of Health*)

In Attendance
Hilary Irons (*Committee Secretary*)

Previous members of the Committee who have contributed to the formulation of these guidelines
* G Dworkin LLB
D R Laurence MD FRCP
R F Mahler MD FRCP
B L Priestly MD FRCP
J P Wight MRCP(UK)

Constitution of the Committee
The Committee on Ethical Issues in Medicine is a standing Committee of the College that advises on the ethics of both research and practice. Membership of the Committee, whilst largely professional, includes non-professional or lay (in relation to medicine) members; members in this category, to whom the College expresses particular thanks, are marked with an asterisk.

ACKNOWLEDGEMENTS

Revision of this document would not have been possible without the commitment and support of the members of the Working Party who devoted their intellect, time and energy to this task. These included Sir Douglas Black (Chairman), Professor Gordon Dunstan, Professor David London, Professor Desmond Laurence and Miss Sue MacGregor. Comments by Rabbi Julia Neuberger and Mrs Claire Foster on the previous edition were also much valued as were the helpful criticisims and comments from the experts we consulted, members of the RCP Committee on Ethical Issues in Medicine and members of Council.

Particular gratitude is extended to Miss Kathy French in Exeter who made several thousand alterations to the text in its myriad drafts, to Hilary Irons at the RCP who co-ordinated the project, to Mrs Claire Foster, Research Fellow at the Centre for Medical Law and Ethics, King's College London, for compiling the index, and to the publications department of the RCP.

DR JOHN TRIPP
Editor

Acknowledgements (previous version)

The Committee on Ethical Issues in Medicine was assisted in its work by a grant from the Nuffield Provincial Hospitals Trust whose support the College gratefully acknowledges.

The College acknowledges the helpful comments of numerous individuals, including Professor Aubrey Diamond and Professor Sir Michael Drury, past President of the Royal College of General Practitioners and Chairman of its Clinical Research Ethics Committee. The College also acknowledges helpful discussion with and opinions received from individuals and organisations too numerous to name, and the extensive literature from this and other countries that has been of enormous assistance.

A Report of the Royal College of P

G
or
ET
in
in s

TH

Published by

THE ROYAL COLLEGE OF PHYSICIANS OF LONDON

AUGUST 1996

Royal College of Physicians of London
11 St Andrews Place, London NW1 4LE

Registered Charity No 210508

ISBN 1 86016 042 5

First printing 1996
Second printing with amendments 1997

Designed and typeset by the Publication Unit of the Royal College of Physicians

Printed in Great Britain by Cathedral Print Services Ltd, Salisbury

CONTENTS

PRESIDENT'S STATEMENT

In 1964 the Medical Research Council published a statement on responsibility in investigations on human subjects. In 1967 the Royal College of Physicians reinforced the Statement by recommending that all research involving patients and normal subjects should undergo ethical review. This led to the establishment of local research ethics committees in National Health Service hospitals — sometimes jointly with university departments. Each committee developed its own method of working and to assist them the College published, in 1984, the first edition on *Guidelines on the practice of ethics committees in medical research*; a second edition followed in 1990.

Recent advances in medical knowledge and technology have opened up new areas for research into health and disease which have led to changes in the public's perception of and attitudes to medical practice and research as well as to some changes in the law. The College has therefore considered it necessary to prepare this third edition of the *Guidelines.*

I hope that these new guidelines will support and inform not only the work of local committees but of other research ethics committees concerned for example with multi-centre research.

The College is aware that the committees often have to make decisions in areas of medicine where there are no hard and fast rules. In some instances the *Guidelines* can do no more than alert ethics committees to special problems; in others, while indicating a generally acceptable course of practice, they deliberately refrain from dictating a 'right' solution. Ultimately, a great deal must depend upon the corporate wisdom of the committees themselves.

While research ethics committees are the custodians of good practice in research, the individual doctor is not absolved from practising the art and science of medicine to the highest standards of medical ethics and of putting forward only those proposals for research which are believed to meet these standards.

August 1996

LESLIE TURNBERG
President, Royal College of Physicians

INTRODUCTION

The first edition of these *Guidelines on the practice of ethics committees in medical research involving human subjects* was prepared by Dr D R Laurence at the request of a steering committee set up by the President of the Royal College of Physicians at the behest of a meeting of chairmen of ethics committees, and others, held at the College in 1982. It was published in 1984.

The document was drafted initially with advice from Drs D A J Tyrell and D W Vere. It was then circulated for comment to the 31 people present at the above meeting and was seen by specialists in a variety of subjects; it was reviewed by some ethics committees. The views of all these, as well as of the Council and a General Meeting of the College, contributed to the document. It was also reviewed by Aubrey Diamond, Professor of Law and then Director of the Institute of Advanced Legal Studies, University of London, who was a member of a research ethics committee.

The *Guidelines* have proved useful, and such has been the interest in ethical issues and developments in medical research that they were revised, in a second edition, under the auspices of the Royal College of Physicians (RCP) Committee on Ethical Issues in Medicine. In 1991 the Department of Health (DoH) issued guidelines to all health authorities confirming that by 1st February 1992 each district health authority (DHA) should have established a local research ethics committee (LREC) with adequate administrative support. The accompanying document *Local research ethics committees* [1] gave guidelines on establishing these committees, identified the ethical principles to which they should have regard and discussed certain special considerations relating to particular groups of research subjects. These guidelines, though brief, conformed closely to the advice given in the second edition of RCP *Guidelines* and we believe that this new edition presents no significant conflict with the DoH document.

CIOMS and WHO have now published International Guidelines on Biomedical Research.[2] Again, we believe that there are no major conflicts between our document and these very important guidelines. There are EU directives in relation to testing of medicines for clinical use and on medical devices with accompanying Good Clinical Practice guidelines and advice for ethics committees.[3]

A compendium of information relevant to research ethics and local research ethics committees was compiled and circulated to all LRECs in 1993.[4] This compendium includes the previous edition of these guidelines as a key document. Most recently the training divison of the Department of Health has circulated an extensive reference

---

1 Department of Health (1991)

2 CIOMS and WHO (1993)

3 EC (1990, 1991, 1993)

4 Foster C G (1993)

booklet on standards for LRECs,[1] a companion booklet on using the standards[2] and a book of standard operating procedures[3].

This new edition of the *Guidelines* is offered as a source of information and opinion on a range of matters concerning the procedures of LRECs. The detail given on some topics, for example consent and liability, is the result of experience of enquiries from individuals and from LRECs. Relevant quotations from documents which, although published, never seem to be at hand when wanted, are also included. It has seemed desirable that practice in the UK should be in accord with international guidelines as far as possible.

Although the *Guidelines* are focussed towards the needs of LRECs and will provide a source of reference for individual members, it is hoped that they will be relevant to the work of all research ethics committees.

To facilitate use in committees, all paragraphs are numbered and a comprehensive index has been provided. As well as the introduction of new information, the text has been substantially re-organised for this edition so that, as far as has been possible, subjects are dealt with under one section heading.

The RCP Committee on Ethical Issues in Medicine will welcome comments and suggestions, particularly from members of LRECs. Correspondence should be addressed to the Honorary Secretary of the Comittee at the College.

---

1 Leigh and Barron Consulting Limited and Christie Associates (1994)

2 Bendall C and Riddell J (1994)

3 Bendall C (1994)

1 PRINCIPLES

Requirements for ethical review

1.1 It is now generally agreed that:

i Research investigations on human beings should conform with codes such as those of the World Medical Association Declaration of Helsinki in its current revision,[1] and of the World Health Organisation (WHO) and its associated bodies;[2]

ii Investigators should not be the sole judges of whether their research does so conform.

These are, however, general statements and do not provide detailed guidance on how the principles which they declare should be applied to individual research proposals, nor how best to organise their independent review.

All medical research subject to review *

1.2 The body (health authority, university, other) that sets up a Local Research Ethics Committee (LREC) should provide that all medical research investigations involving human subjects, including the use of fetal material, embryos, and tissue from the recently dead (which pose similar ethical problems), should come before it. Optional or selective submission, which has been practised in some institutions and health districts, cannot be justified.

1.3 The Department of Health (DoH) requires all projects undertaken by NHS staff, carried out on NHS premises, involving participants via the NHS or involving access to past or present NHS records to be reviewed by an LREC.[3]

1.4 The DoH issued a formal guideline (HSG(91)5) in 1991 stating that district health authorities (DHAs) are responsible for establishing LRECs 'to advise National Health Service (NHS) bodies on the ethical acceptability of research proposals involving human subjects'. The Medical Research Council (MRC) and other bodies that fund or authorise research, eg NHS regional R&D directorates etc, require ethical review of projects before making a grant, and most scientific journals require it as a condition of publication. The MRC has published a series of useful booklets.[4]

Objectives of research ethics committees

Facilitating good research

1.5 The objectives of RECs are to maintain ethical standards of practice in research, to protect subjects of research from harm, to preserve the subjects' rights and to provide reassurance to the public that this is being done.

---

* But see 6.22–6.24

1 World Medical Association (1989)

2 CIOMS and WHO (1993)

3 Department of Health (1991)

4 MRC (1985; 1991a,b,c,d)

1.6 In achieving these objectives, RECs should remember that good research benefits patients and society and that they should take care not to hinder it without good cause.

1.7 RECs may also protect research workers and institutions from unjustified criticism.

1.8 Subject always to adequate safeguards, patients should not be denied the opportunity to help in the advancement of medical knowledge.

Respect for persons

1.9 Respect for persons referred to in the Declaration of Helsinki and the CIOMS/WHO guidelines includes respect for an individual's capacity to make reasoned decisions, and protection of those whose capacity is impaired or who are in some way dependent or vulnerable.

Ethical obligations

1.10 Clinical investigators have an ethical obligation to maximise benefits and minimise harms and wrongs. This principle demands that the risks of research are reasonable in relation to expected benefits, that the research design is sound and that the investigators are competent, both to conduct the research and to safeguard the welfare of research participants.

1.11 They have also an ethical obligation to treat each person in accordance with what is morally right and proper and to achieve an equitable distribution of both burdens and benefits of participation in research. The CIOMS/WHO guidelines include the following paragraph:

> 'Research involving human subjects should be carried out only by, or strictly supervised by, suitably qualified and experienced investigators and in accordance with a protocol that clearly states:
>
> - the aim of the research;
> - the reasons for proposing that it involves human subjects;
> - the nature and degree of any known risks to the subjects;
> - the means proposed for ensuring that subjects' consent will be adequately informed and voluntary.
>
> The protocol should be scientifically and ethically appraised by one or more suitably constituted review bodies, independent of the investigators.'

Patient–doctor relationship

1.12 The patient–doctor relationship is based on the understanding that the doctor is concerned to put the interest of the individual patient first. Patients generally believe this and it is essential that their confidence should not be impaired. Research may involve subjugation of this interest. The nature and extent of this must be clearly known to and understood by participants. Lack of truthfulness or frankness about research on the grounds, for example, that the research is 'harmless' and that consent need not be obtained because the process of obtaining it 'will cause needless anxiety', is a breach of this relationship.

Knowledge of involvement

1.13 It is a general rule that people who are subjects of research, whether they be healthy or sick, should be made clearly aware of their position and of the nature of the research (see 7.18–7.30). Any investigator who proposes to depart from this rule should be prepared to justify the procedure before an REC or even in a court of law.

Clinical responsibility

1.14 Clinical responsibility for all patients in the NHS (and usually in private practice) ultimately falls on consultants and/or on their general practitioners. GPs and consultants, to whom the information is relevant, should be informed when research is conducted with their patients by their colleagues or by others. Sometimes a patient is attended by more than one consultant, eg surgeon and anaesthetist. In such cases the consultant who is responsible for the *overall care* of the patient should always be involved alongside any others.

Consent

1.15 A principle of the Declaration of Helsinki is that subjects' consent to their participation in research must be voluntary. To ensure that this consent is valid participants must be sufficiently informed about the research (as above) and have adequate time to make an unpressured decision. Consent must normally be recorded by the subject's signature on an appropriate form (see 7.31–7.49).

Voluntary withdrawal

1.16 In addition to ensuring that subjects are informed and have given consent, every effort should be made to ensure that subjects have an opportunity to comment and ask questions and that they can, if they wish, easily withdraw from a research investigation without giving reasons and without incurring any penalty or alteration in their relationship with those giving medical care (see 7.38).

The current status of LRECs

1.17 LRECs are now well established. The enormous amount of continuing medical research has given them a volume and variety of experience that is probably not equalled in other areas of research involving human subjects.

1.18 Such information as the College has suggests a general raising of standards and increasing conformity in the practice of LRECs. This has been helped by common acceptance of authoritative guidelines, by training of members and also by the meetings of LREC chairmen held at the RCP with the support of the DoH. Nevertheless, the King's Fund inquiry/survey[1] confirms that the practice of LRECs continues to be variable, not only due to natural differences of opinion, but due to disagreement about, and sometimes even unawareness of, what issues fall within the scope of ethical review. In particular, there may be discrepancies between institutions where research is an occasional or minor activity and those where it is a frequent and major activity. There have been suggestions that the structure, function and methods of working of LRECs should be subject to statutory control. The DoH formal guidance, although not in itself a statutory control, would carry authority in any legal proceedings.

---

1 Neuberger J (1992)

Populations and institutions served by LRECs

1.19 Most LRECs are constituted to serve an NHS district health commission (DHC) rather than a single institution. This means that committees may cover several institutions as well as general practice. The committee's prime responsibility is to research subjects and thus the fact that it is appointed by an authority with public health responsibility such as a DHC is appropriate.

1.20 In some centres there is a single LREC for all research on humans, set up jointly, where appropriate, by a health commission and university. In other centres there is a committee of the health commission that reviews research on patients and also a committee of the university or medical school that would review research initiated by university staff. There is no reason of principle to prefer one arrangement to the other.

1.21 General practitioners are independent contractors either as fundholders or in District Health Commissions. Arrangements should be made for research in general practice to be put before an LREC as required by the DoH.[1]

Committees serving individual specialties or clinical areas

1.22 RECs need a sufficient body of work to develop the ethos and the skills to apply ethical principles to research in human subjects. In general, it is not appropriate for medical specialties or individual Trusts to seek to set up their own committees. A desirable feature of RECs is that specialists should have to persuade their peers experienced in other areas, as well as lay people, that what they propose is acceptable. Nevertheless, the fears of specialists that an REC will not understand their research deserve consideration and this can be met by co-option to the committee or, according to circumstances, by the formation of a sub-committee with over-lapping membership. Some areas of particular ethical difficulty have resulted in the setting up of national committees to consider research and, often, practice in these fields of research. These include the DoH Gene Therapy Advisory Committee (GTAC), and the Human Fertilisation and Embryology Authority (HFEA).

1.23 Research ethics committees set up by independent contract research companies or by pharmaceutical or other industrial companies to review the testing of their own products (particularly relevant and seen as necessary by many companies for Phase I healthy volunteer studies (see A1.1–A1.3)), pose particular problems of obtaining members whose independence and credibility are publicly assured. These problems have been addressed by the Association for the British Pharmaceutical Industry (ABPI).[2] Approval by such committees does not give exemption from appropriate submission to LRECs.

1.24 For Phase IV trials (see A1.6) which are of licensed medicines, frequently large scale, and which may be perceived as having a promotional purpose, the ABPI recommends the setting up of a steering committee with a preponderance of non-company (and presumably non-investigator) members.[3]

---

1 Department of Health (1991)

2 ABPI (1994)

3 ABPI (1993a)

Where there is no committee

1.25 If there is no ethics committee, eg in a school, factory or office, the investigators should approach the NHS LREC which should be willing to consider proposals, even though they do not involve NHS patients or staff.

2 TERMS OF REFERENCE OF LRECs

Duties of an LREC

2.1 An LREC should:

- advise its appointing authority on all matters pertaining to the ethics of research involving human subjects;
- review proposals for research to be carried out in the institutions or area of that authority;
- review proposals for research to be carried out by staff of the authority in other places where there is no ethics committee. *Note:* Where the other place has an ethics committee, the committee of the investigator's own institution need not necessarily be involved;
- not undertake functions that might conflict with the above, for example, it should not act as a research funding or grant-giving committee;
- make an annual, or more frequent, report to the appointing authority, which should be made available to the public (see 5.20);
- be prepared to inform the Medicines Control Agency of the DoH (MCA) of applications which are refused on grounds relating to licensing or safety issues.

Scientific quality

2.2 The nature of the decision that an LREC has to make is largely defined above; but the question of the extent to which scientific quality, design and conduct should be considered continues to cause difficulty. Badly planned, poorly designed research that causes inconvenience to subjects and may carry risk, is unethical. Plainly, a highly rigorous scientific evaluation is beyond the capacity of the great majority of LRECs. Nonetheless, they should approve only studies which are of good quality. Most committees will do their best in this area, using their own knowledge and knowledge of their colleagues, but they should not hesitate to make use of external advisers for difficult problems, particularly in the areas of design and statistical evaluation of protocols. Where peer review has been carried out by an expert committee of a funding body such as the MRC, this should normally be accepted as evidence of scientific validity.

2.3 Where a committee is doubtful of the scientific quality and/or risk evaluation, it should tell the applicant to obtain expert advice. A committee should not reject an application on grounds of low scientific quality unless it has satisfied itself that it has adequate knowledge and expert advice to justify this step.

Student research

2.4 RECs may receive requests from students of medicine or paramedical disciplines, many of whose courses require them to undertake a piece of research. It is proper that students should be trained in research and that, where appropriate, this training should include making an application to an REC. Although much student research cannot be expected to produce significant benefit for the subject or for mankind in general, it is nevertheless appropriate to invite subjects to participate in such research since the training of students is in itself of benefit to mankind. In assessing such student research, the committee will be aware that the risk-benefit equation must be applied so that such research will not normally carry more than minimal risk (see 7.2).

2.5 Subjects must be given full information about the purpose of the research for the education of students.

Investigators and premises

2.6 An REC will wish to be satisfied that the investigators have sufficient clinical and personal skills (or adequate supervision) and that the research will be carried out in appropriate professional premises. These considerations will give confidence that the dignity of patients will be respected and that the possibility of unforseen danger is minimised.

Ethics of clinical practice

2.7 From time to time an REC is approached by a clinician with an ethical problem of medical practice (not of research). LRECs are not constituted for this purpose, and it is unwise for a committee to respond formally to requests that are outside its terms of reference, though members may well agree to engage in informal discussion. The College recognises the importance of these issues and the need to develop a means of handling such requests. Accreditation standards for hospitals suggested by the King's Fund include the existence of mechanisms to consider ethical issues and implement policies.[1]

Scientific fraud

2.8 An REC may or may not be the most appropriate body to investigate allegations of scientific fraud. If it hears of such an allegation and believes that it requires investigation, the committee should attempt to deal with it at local level, for example through the Dean of of the relevant medical school or other appropriate authority. Where this is impracticable or inappropriate, it should ensure that information is passed to a more appropriate body, for example, the Conference of Medical Royal Colleges or one of its constituent bodies. This College has produced a report on fraud and misconduct in medical research[2] and is setting up a standing committee to consider these issues.

Termination of research

2.9 Ethical issues are not confined to the question whether to start a research project. They can include when to stop; for example, in order to avoid needlessly pro-

---

1 King's Fund hospital accreditation programme 1994/1995

2 Royal College of Physicians (1991)

longed use of a less effective treatment, a therapeutic trial in a serious condition should be so constructed as to provide for interim or sequential analysis as the trial progresses. Note that interim or sequential analysis requires specialist statistical advice.[1] Trials should not be terminated simply because of a commercial interest.

2.10 REC approval should be time limited and applicants should, therefore, state a period in their original application for which they expect the research to continue. This time may be extended by chairman's action where appropriate.

Adverse events

2.11 Serious adverse events* should be promptly reported to the REC by investigators who should be made aware of this duty in the letter from the committee when giving approval. In trials involving drugs or novel equipment and trials sponsored by industry, such reporting to the sponsor is in any case mandatory under *Good clinical (research) practice guidelines*.[2] Such research is also formally audited[3] and medicines research must be so under EU guidelines.[4] Reports should be copied to the REC who should also be made aware of adverse event reports from other participating centres or other trials of a drug. In the latter instance, it is helpful to have a commentary or interpretation of the significance of adverse events by the local investigator.

Other monitoring

2.12 Plainly it is impracticable, even if it were desirable, for an REC to monitor in detail the conduct of ongoing investigations, but Committees should not lose contact with any investigations they have approved.

2.13 Some form of follow-up is desirable, if only an annual questionnaire to applicants. It should establish whether the project has been completed, abandoned (the reason should be given) or is still in progress in the original or other form approved by the committee. Investigators may be asked to send reprints of publications to the committee.

2.14 It has been suggested that RECs should undertake more detailed follow-up and monitoring of projects. For example, in order to satisfy themselves that informed consent has been given by participants in a project, they may occasionally check how information is given to patients and how consent is obtained. This would clearly be impracticable for all projects, but a committee might decide to do detailed follow up on selected projects.

---

* A serious adverse event is any event associated with a life threatening or long-term complication or one which might affect the integrity of the study

1 McPherson K (1974)

2 ABPI (1992)

3 ABPI (1993b)

4 EU (1990)

2.15 It has been suggested that a sample of patients should be asked, after participating in a study, for their views on the research and its outcome for them. We are not aware of any reported experience of this being done or of its value.

Publication

2.16 Most reputable journals require authors to confirm that their clinical research has been approved by REC when they submit it for publication.

2.17 It is unacceptable in principle that an investigator should agree to conditions that may prohibit or impair the possibility of publication, though some delay may sometimes be acceptable. This applies whether the sponsor of the research is a pharmaceutical company, a government department or any other agency. Investigators should agree a publication policy in advance and include it in their application.[1]

2.18 It has been suggested that RECs should ensure that, where possible, negative results of studies are published. Meta-analyses of research studies suffer from the difficulty that only positive results tend to be published unless the investigator is looking for a negative result. In the case of drug trials, this means that studies which do not have an outcome that supports the use of a drug may not be published, and this may bias the literature. While ensuring publication of negative results is beyond the role or ability of RECs, it is important that they do ensure that publication of such results is not precluded in advance or otherwise impeded by sponsors in order to safeguard their own interests.

Costs of research

2.19 If routine health services, eg beds, pharmacy, radiology, haematology, clinical chemistry, endoscopy, are required for research, then it is appropriate for the LREC to check with the investigator that arrangements have been agreed with the providers of the service. This is often achieved by requesting the signature of an appropriate person, eg relevant hospital clinical director or the senior partner in a general practice.

2.20 Although the allocation of resources has ethical implications, consideration of this is an issue for NHS management. Those who distribute resources will generally require that a project has the approval of an REC before considering it for support. The fact of approval does not carry any implication that resources ought to be provided and REC approval should not be used to assert this.

2.21 It has been suggested that LRECs should promote research in areas of priority to the NHS but this is clearly outside their remit (see 1.5–1.6)

2.22 The REC's adjudication of the ethics of a research protocol should not take into account that the results of medical, social or environmental research might later give rise to demands for implementation that may be expensive, though, of course, such matters are of legitimate ethical concern to those responsible for allocating scarce resources.

---

1 ABPI (1988)

3 RESPONSIBILITIES IN LAW

Statute and common law

3.1 The public will reasonably expect research involving human subjects to be conducted in accordance with the law. It is not easy to envisage circumstances where an REC would approve a research project that infringed the law, eg Medicines Act, Mental Health Act, Data Protection Act. It may sometimes be appropriate for a committee to ask an investigator to confirm that a study complies with the law; this may involve obtaining legal advice.

Liability of appointing authority

3.2 The authority appointing an REC (health authority, university, other) may be either directly liable or vicariously liable for the acts of members of RECs, according to whether they are employees or non-employees of the authority.

Duty of care

3.3 The issues have not been tested in the courts, but RECs and the authorities appointing them almost certainly owe a duty of care to research subjects that imposes upon them the obligation to take reasonable care to protect their interests. Failure to do so could lead to claims for negligence, although the likelihood of a successful claim against members of a well conducted REC is remote. The DoH expects the appointing authority to ensure appropriate membership and proper working practices.

Claims against committee members

3.4 Exposure to claims is likely to come only from research subjects who allege they were injured by a failure on the part of members of the committee to identify the risks of the research in circumstances where any reasonable REC would have identified them, or have insisted that the subject be appropriately warned or that the research be dropped.

3.5 As a result of publicity concerning the compensation arrangements made by industrial companies sponsoring research, there is now a general expectation by volunteers (patient or healthy) that in the event of injury caused by participation in non-therapeutic research or in therapeutic research using novel treatments or medicines for unlicensed indications, compensation will be paid independent of proof of negligence. Where no provision for compensation has been made this is a material fact which ought to be disclosed to the research subject by the investigator, and, where there is risk to the subject, an REC should ensure that subjects are made aware of their position in regard to compensation arrangements or the lack of these[1] (see 9.26).

---

1 Department of Health (1991) Paragraph 3.20

3.6 Members conduct their activities as individuals: the committee is not incorporated, ie it has no separate legal personality, and so cannot be sued as an entity. Where an allegation of negligence against committee members is proven, then it is possible that members will be personally liable in respect of their own expertise.

Indemnification of committee members

3.7 The College advises that LRECs should approach the appointing organisation (health authority, university or other) with the request that it should formally agree to indemnify committee members for loss arising out of the exercise of their function. Indemnity should include the costs of legal representation (which may in itself be considerable even in a case where the claim is later dropped) as well as any compensation that may ultimately be awarded to the research subject. New members should be advised as to their position in relation to this and may wish to reconsider their participation in the absence of such an undertaking.

4 MEMBERSHIP OF LRECs

Principles

4.1 Members need to be people of goodwill, with a high regard for the human personality, for truthfulness and for the continued advance of science in the interest of society. Those who are totally opposed to research investigations or experiments on humans should be left to oppose the system from outside and should not be invited on to the committee. On the other hand, individuals who are acquiescent and may be thought likely to give automatic approval are also not suitable members. A majority of the medical members should be mainly employed in providing clinical care.

4.2 Among the members there should be individuals other than professional investigators who will look at applications critically from the subject's point of view, and this role may be taken by a number of different individuals, particularly nurses and lay members.

4.3 For the community to have confidence in LRECs their membership should be seen to be broad and not exclusively medical; and the lay members to be persons of responsibility and standing who will not be overawed by medical members.

4.4 Lay members have a particular role in relation to issues of consent and the clarity of information given to subjects.

Information for regulatory authorities

4.5 A list of the names and status of the members of an LREC is sometimes sought by a pharmaceutical company to meet a requirement of the USA Food and Drug Administration to which the company is making application. There is no reason to refuse this.

Membership

4.6 Membership of an LREC should normally be constituted as follows:

Medical members. These will include both those chiefly occupied with clinical care and experienced clinical investigators; a general practitioner should be included.

Non-medical research workers. According to the types of research coming before the committee these will include, for example, psychologists, social scientists, social workers.

Nurses. At least one nurse should be included, preferably in active practice with patients.

Lay members. At least two persons not practising or trained in any medical or paramedical discipline should sit on the committee. At least one lay member should be independent of the institution or the health authority served by the committee. A lay member with legal training can be of great value but the role should be a general one, not solely to answer questions of law. A legal member should not be the professional adviser to the appointing authority.

Both sexes should be represented on the committee and amongst the lay members.

4.7 The DoH state that the sponsoring authority will appoint the chairman and vice-chairman but may do so after consultation with the committee (see 4.10).

4.8 The committee should be of manageable size, eg not more than 12. Although it may be attractive to consider the appointment of alternates for absent members, we believe that this compromises the effective working of a committee and where possible, membership should be arranged so that where a member having a particular skill or affiliation is regarded as essential for a quorum (see 5.17), membership in this category should be duplicated.

Specialist representation

4.9 It is not practicable to include specialists in all the fields, medical and allied, that may have a scientific or other input to all the various proposals that may come before it. The reasonable requests by specialists that members of their specialty should always be involved in assessing their applications, or at least where there is a possibility of rejection, can be met by having two members of that discipline on the committee where applications are frequent. Alternatively, in other appropriate recurrent or occasional cases, specialist needs can be met by co-option or by formation of a subcommittee, permanent or *ad hoc*, with overlapping membership.

Chairman

4.10 While most LRECs are chaired by a medical person many are now chaired by a lay person and the value of having a lay chairman for meetings is recognised. Most lay people will, however, need professional advice to inform effective 'chairman's action' (see 5.10–5.13) and it may then be helpful to have a medically qualified vice-chairman or secretary with powers to take such action. DoH guidelines state that either the chairman or vice-chairman should be lay.

Appointments

4.11 The responsible authority, eg district health authority, academic executive, will formally appoint the LREC members, having taken appropriate advice including advice from representative lay organisations such as community health councils, patient organisations etc. An established committee, knowing its own needs, may propose appropriate names. The appointment of lay members may need wider consultation than the appointment of professional members. It is not appropriate to construct an LREC by inviting and accepting nominations from a range of bodies claiming an interest.

4.12 It is essential that members should serve on the committee as individuals and not as delegates taking instruction from other bodies or reporting to them.

4.13 The committee will report to the appointing authority, though details of its consideration of applications will be confidential.

Duration of membership

4.14 Duration of membership should be prescribed (for example, 3 to 5 years which may be renewed once). It should be remembered that although the committee should not stagnate, members need time to absorb the ethos and to develop the skills of ethical review and that it is also important not to lose a valuable and willing member simply because time has passed. This applies particularly to lay members who may not be as easily replaced as are professional members.

New members and training

4.15 New members should be encouraged to undertake one of the courses available regionally and nationally for new members probably after they have attended two or three meetings. All members should be provided with some core material including the DoH documents and these and other guidelines referred to elsewhere (see Introduction, p1–2). They should also have ready access to a wide range of literature such as is contained in the King's College, London *Manual for Research Ethics Committees* [1] and other specialist material such as that listed in the bibliography.

Update

4.16 It is important to circulate to the committee relevant publications on general policy and on particular aspects, such as consent for research involving children, that appear from time to time. The chairman or other member having a particular interest may undertake the selection.

---

1 Foster C G (1993)

5 METHOD OF WORKING

Administrative support

5.1 A committee serving a health district or university will need substantial administrative, including secretarial, help. This must be provided by the appointing authorities.

Consideration of applications

5.2 Some RECs may do their work entirely at meetings.

5.3 Applicants may be invited to attend meetings, either routinely (impractical for most committees) or for specific reasons. Such reasons might include the need for the committee to meet the applicant, the need to clarify the proposal or to allow the best opportunity for an applicant to answer questions raised by the committee.

5.4 Although the applicant may be present for discussion of the project, the committee may wish to make its decision in private.

5.5 Some applications raise only minor ethical issues and some committees arrange for these applications to be circulated so that comments may be received; the application can thus be provisionally and expeditiously approved without convening an unnecessary meeting. The size of the workload is obviously relevant to these choices. A disadvantage of working by post is that committee meetings may become so rare that the valuable mutual exchanges between members are lost, and lay members particularly will feel isolated. It is, therefore, unacceptable to seek to conduct all business without meetings.

5.6 To work entirely or almost entirely by mail or by chairman's action, even if decisions are later put before a meeting, is also unacceptable. Reasonably frequent meetings are essential to allow a committee ethos to develop.

Quorum

5.7 It is useful to define the size and membership of a quorum. This should normally include at least one lay person, a general practitioner, a research oriented doctor and a member of each sex.

Full review by an REC

5.8 Most projects will require formal review by the REC.

Decisions

5.9 Decisions made by consensus will be preferred by most committees if at all possible. The size of a required majority should be decided in advance for those occasions when general agreement is not attainable; the majority may be qualified by the necessity to include at least one lay member. Prudence should guide the chairman if, in a particular case, a majority decision would leave consciences with reasonable ground for serious misgiving.

Chairman's action

5.10 Investigations that pose no ethical problems, and are without risk of distress or injury, psychological or physical, to the subjects, eg some epidemiology, some surveys of the public's eating or smoking habits, assessment of patient information and education, should nevertheless be the subject of an application but may be expeditiously handled by chairman's action.

5.11 The LREC could thus arrange for the chairman or deputy, alone or sometimes in consultation with another member, to receive a proposal and, where appropriate, expeditiously to issue provisional approval on its behalf, always reporting these approvals to the next meeting for ratification. Where the chairman is not satisfied that an investigation falls into this class, the applicant should be told that an application for full committee review is required.

5.12 Rarely, chairman's approval may be given solely because of urgency, eg where a clinician wishes to enter a patient into a clinical trial because it is believed that this is the best treatment option. Wherever there is doubt, an application should go to the full committee.

5.13 Sometimes an application for a study judged by the chairman not to require ethical review is put forward because a research funding body has a rule that it will not consider an application unless it is accompanied by evidence of ethics committee approval. Chairmen may give such 'approval' expeditiously without standing on the niceties of the situation. Even where there is an ethical issue a chairman may judge that this will be resolvable and approve 'in principle', but subject to later full committee approval after the decision to fund the research is made; this saves the committee from reviewing proposals that are never proceeded with. The research funding organisation should be informed of this procedure which is acceptable to many, including the MRC. Time constraints may result in the need for the two approvals to proceed together where there is expectation of funding approval.

Class approvals

5.14 Individual investigators or departments that conduct ongoing research which varies in detail but conforms to the same general pattern (for example, some programmes in epidemiology or in training students), may be given a 'class' approval to avoid repetitive submissions of projects differing only in detail. This is particularly appropriate for projects that pose no risk of distress or injury to subjects. All such projects should be individually reported to the committee, and papers submitted for chairman's perusal and reference to the committee where appropriate. This process may also be used for studies in which a local investigator may or may not be involved (see 6.20–6.21).

Unapproved proposals

5.15 Experience has shown that although it is rare for a project to be found totally unacceptable, it is common for projects to be modified following discussion with a committee. If a proposal is not approved, the reasons should be given to the applicant in writing. Investigators should be made aware that they are entitled to have an adverse decision reviewed and to make written and/or oral representations to the committee. In situations of particular difficulty, the REC might, on the request of an investigator, appoint referees by mutual agreement or ask the appropriate Royal College to do so.

Availability for consultation

5.16 Committees should make it known that investigators planning research may seek advice from the committee or from a member.

Sanctions

5.17 RECs have no direct sanctions, but if they discover that their advice is unheeded or that clinical investigations are being conducted without reference to them, they should report the facts to the body that set them up, eg an NHS health commission or hospital or a university board and, if appropriate, to professional organisations such as Royal Colleges and the GMC. NHS employees and general practitioners are effectively subject to the Department of Health guidelines on LRECs which make clear that all research involving patients must be submitted to a properly constituted LREC. Though these guidelines do not apply directly to research undertaken outside the NHS, committees have a responsibility to make other employers/authorities aware of medical research which is not being conducted within this safeguard. Plainly, an investigator who bypasses or ignores the recommendations of a properly authorised REC could be vulnerable to professional disciplinary or even legal proceedings.

5.18 Where a committee is dissatisfied with the conduct of an investigation it may withdraw approval already given. It should then inform the applicant that approval has been withdrawn. The investigation, if it is still in progress, should cease forthwith and the investigator shall not thereafter claim that the research had ethical approval.

Protocol amendments

5.19 Amendments to investigation protocols should be approved by RECs, and investigators reminded that approval is restricted to the protocol as submitted until any amendments are approved.

Reports

5.20 RECs should report annually to the authorities that set them up. In addition to a list of members, number of meetings and any other obviously relevant matter, it should include a list of the titles of projects approved (whether in their original form or after modification) and it should include those that are not approved or are later withdrawn. This College believes that this latter group should be listed but not referred to by title or investigator. The report should be available for inspection by the public.

Confidentiality

5.21 Confidentiality of REC proceedings (as distinct from decisions) should be preserved because the issues considered are often complicated and delicate. Uninformed or unbalanced publicity could arouse emotions that are damaging to all concerned, especially to patients; moreover some investigators who have had an original idea fear that this may be passed to others who are in competition with them. Minutes of LRECs should be available to the chairmen of the appointing authorities.

Declaration of interest

5.22 Just as applicants should declare any interest (see 10.1–10.2), so members of an REC should declare their interests, for example, where an application relates to testing a product of a company to which the member is an adviser or where the member conducts (competitive) research in the same field. The chairman will decide whether the interest disqualifies the member from the discussion. Where the chairman has an interest, a vice-chairman should take the chair.

Adverse events

5.23 Serious adverse events affecting research subjects should be reported promptly to the committee which should satisfy itself that a proper enquiry is conducted and consider the implications for the continuation of the research.

Access to the REC

5.24 Direct access to the REC should be available to research subjects who are dissatisfied. When this happens it should be the responsibility of investigators to inform research subjects.

Fees

5.25 In the case of direct applications from the private medical sector or other non-NHS source, a handling charge may be made, but it should cover no more than the relevant administration costs of the REC and is often waived for universities, charities and similar institutions.

5.26 Members either should not be paid (other than reimbursement of expenses or loss of earnings) or, if they receive an honorarium it should be modest and should not be paid by any body with a financial interest in the outcome of applications. The work of some committees is becoming increasingly onerous for both professional and lay members. Although there is a widely held view that it is inappropriate for members to be paid on the basis that this is a public service, it seems likely that the increasing workload will mean that at least officers will require payment for work which may take up one or more sessions of time per week. It would be counter-productive if the burden of work discouraged people from serving on RECs.

6 MEDICAL RESEARCH

6.1 Medical research is a broad world-wide activity. Its two main objectives are to increase and refine the body of knowledge on which that part of the practice of medicine which is science-based depends; and to explore the practical ways in which that knowledge can be applied in the prevention and treatment of disease. Increased knowledge can come from studies at all levels of biological organisation, from sub-cellular compounds and particles to whole organisms, both individual and grouped in defined populations. While the direct responsibility of RECs may be centred on the 'applied' component of medical research, and perhaps largely on the numerous trials of the efficacy and safety of medicines, it should be appreciated that investigations on patients and on people in normal health have substantially contributed to basic medical knowledge and to the advantage of patients and the community.

6.2 Medical research may be conducted both on patients and on healthy people. In this document all research involving patients, and some, but not all, research involving people who are not patients, is considered as medical research. For example drug studies on healthy volunteers and some research on healthy living or training exercises, are considered as medical research whether conducted by doctors, nurses, paramedical, psychological or community based investigators. These *Guidelines* are applicable to studies carried out by students in their professional education and some types of audit (see below).

Definition and classes of research

6.3 The definition of research continues to present difficulties.

Medical research and innovative medical practice

6.4 The distinction between medical research and innovative medical practice derives from the *intent.* In medical *practice* the sole intention is to benefit the *individual patient* consulting the clinician, not to gain knowledge of general benefit, though such knowledge may emerge from the clinical experience gained.* In medical *research* the primary intention is to advance knowledge so that *patients in general* may benefit: the individual patient may or may not benefit directly.

6.5 When a clinician departs in a significant way from standard or accepted practice entirely for the benefit of a particular individual patient, and with the patient's consent, the innovation need not constitute research, though it may be described as an experiment in the sense that it is novel and unvalidated.† Clinicians should be prepared to justify their innovative therapy both ethically and scientifically if challenged.

* For example, a randomised and blinded multiple crossover trial of one or two treatments for a single patient may appear initially to be research but is in fact medical practice. See Irwig, Glaziou and March (1995) for a discussion of trials which may be either medical practice or research.

† In this context, an 'experiment' is a procedure adopted on the chance of its succeeding. 'Research' is a systematic experiment or series of observations to establish facts or principles and generalisable knowledge.

6.6 Extension of such an experiment into wider use or general application should, *prima facie*, be regarded as research.

6.7 The blurring of this distinction has given rise to published correspondence.[1] Clinicians involved in sensitive areas of innovative practice (eg *in vitro* fertilisation, see 8.32–8.34) may wish to conduct such practice as descriptive or qualitative research so allowing them to put their protocol before an LREC. The distinction between innovative therapy and research may be clarified by an appropriate medical member of the committee being available for consultation by clinicians.

Medical or clinical audit and research

6.8 Audit has been defined in a number of ways. It is the investigation of clinical practice and institutional systems, usually against a given or accepted standard. The distinction from research has been defined as follows: 'Research is finding out what you ought to be doing; audit is seeing whether you are doing what you ought to be doing'.*

6.9 In contrast to audit, research concerns the scientific investigation of a predicted but not necessarily proven relationship between or among variables.

6.10 Some observational studies of outcomes for patients may also be described as audit, even though they may not provide feedback for remedial action.

6.11 It has been agreed (eg DoH guidelines) that such activity does not require approval of an LREC. In practice, such investigations may involve not only scrutiny of patients' notes, but interviews with patients, or even the relatives of deceased patients. Such activity clearly may be intrusive and if so, might properly be assessed by research ethics committees. Where there is doubt it may, therefore, be appropriate to submit audit projects, to the chairman of an REC for a decision as to whether this should be considered by the committee or classed as audit not requiring review.

Classes of research

There are two major classes of research:

i that which involves making observations *without any direct interference* with the subject (un-intrusive or non-invasive), such as research involving the use of personal medical records alone (see 6.22–6.24);

ii that which involves *interference with the subject* (psychological intrusion, including intrusion on privacy, or physical invasion). Such interference, psychological or physical, raises ethical issues which whether large or small should be subject to ethical review.

6.12 Research may also be classed as: (a) interventions which may benefit the individual participant *(therapeutic research)* and (b) interventions which are unlikely to benefit the individual participant *(non-therapeutic research)*.

6.13 It is sometimes urged that because a participant in a randomised controlled therapeutic trial (commonly offered as an example of therapeutic research) may

* Quoted as an adage by Dr Anthony Hopkins in correspondence regarding these guidelines.

1 Chalmers I and Chalmers T C (1990)

be allocated to placebo or dummy treatment, such studies cannot reasonably be described as 'therapeutic'. While there is substance in this, a patient in the placebo arm may benefit by being offered the treatment if the result of the trial favours treatment. Nevertheless the general distinction of 'therapeutic' and 'non-therapeutic' research is useful.

Research using standard or conventional treatments

6.14 Some studies involve the randomisation of patients to one, two, or more standard treatments. Clinicians have suggested that provided they take due care to prevent randomisation of any patient for whom there might be a clinical or personal (patient) preference for one treatment over another, there is no need for ethical review. Such studies do, however, present ethical issues and should be put before an REC which may agree that explicit patient consent is inappropriate but may, nevertheless, consider that patients are entitled to know that they are participating in research.

Multi-location studies

6.15 Multi-location studies are increasingly undertaken in epidemiological and clinical practice and in pharmaceutical research. Currently, some such studies are impeded because of the necessity to submit studies for approval by LRECs in all locations where participants are recruited, living or are treated. While it remains policy that all such research projects should be approved by these LRECs we believe that urgent steps must be taken to expedite this process. Standardisation of the format of application forms would assist considerably (see 11.3).

A central research ethics committee(s)

6.16 We support the setting up of a central research ethics committee(s) to consider multi-location research. Its membership needs to command professional and lay respect and should be competent to take decisions and approve the research in relation to purpose, scientific merit, risk/benefit issues, methodology (including statistics) subject information, consent procedures and overall design.

6.17 LRECs should then be asked to accept this (part) approval and specifically consider locally relevant issues such as appropriateness of research personnel, premises, language of patient information sheets and consent forms and give an expeditious local decision. Concerns about the issues considered by the central committee should be raised with them rather than with the investigator.

6.18 The Royal College of General Practitioners has for some years had a clinical research ethics committee to review multi-location studies in general practice. Applicants to this committee are informed that studies which have been approved need also to be submitted to local research ethics committees by local investigators. LRECs will consider the appropriateness of investigators, premises, the content of patient information sheets and consent forms but only exceptionally consider problems in relation to the scientific content or general ethical issues.

6.19 The Department of Health has recently published a Consultation Paper based on a CMO working party with proposals for multi-location RECs (MRECs). It is proposed that an MREC should be based in each English region and suggested that similar arrangements might be made for single committees in Wales and Scotland, with LRECs in Northern Ireland relying on a mainland MREC. The proposals are broadly consistent with the above paragraphs (6.16–6.18). It is suggested that projects where more than five LRECs are involved might be referred to an MREC. Each MREC would be empowered to consider the science and ethics of a proposal on behalf of all LRECs involved in any region.

Studies recruiting few or no local patients

6.20 Another class of research which has caused difficulty for LRECs and investigator is the type of national (or international) study that recruits patients with rare conditions. The commonest examples are:

Cancer and leukaemia protocols where in any one district the number of possible protocols that *might* be used is large but because of the rarity of the conditions few will ever be used.

Studies which 'collect' cases of rare conditions for research. The British Paediatric Association Surveillance Unit runs a number of such studies for many of which most districts will never recruit patients.

6.21 A pragmatic solution is proposed as follows: the originators of the proposal or a key investigator should present the protocol to a single REC.* If granted approval from this committee the investigator should suggest the following strategy to participating clinicians. Clinicians who may enter patients into such trials should seek a 'class approval' (see 5.14) for the type of studies they may undertake. When entering a patient the clinician will be supplied with a protocol information sheet and consent form which should be used in the usual way, but afterwards notifying their own LREC that they have entered a patient, supplying a copy of relevant material, if required and confirming to them that the protocol has been approved by a named REC.

Unintrusive research

6.22 Most guidelines[1] state that all medical research, including the use of anonymous or confidentially kept records, must be subject to review by an independent REC (though see 8.24–8.27 in relation to subject consent.) This advice has implications for other groups such as non-medical bodies conducting research in, for example, nutrition and the social sciences.

6.23 A working party with a strong lay membership concluded that to require formal ethical review of research involving personal medical records or stored biological samples alone is likely to delay or even inhibit valuable research: they further recommended, provided that such research is carried out with scrupulous confidentiality, it is by its nature harmless and does not require submission to an LREC. Council of the RCP approved this report and agreed to publish it to facilitate wider discussion; it is summarised in Appendix B and has been published in full.[2]

---

* Ideally this committee will be one which has experience of the consideration of similar protocols.

1 These include CIOMS and WHO (1993),Department of Health (1991; 1994), MRC (1985; 1992) and Bendall (1994), though Leigh and Barron Consulting Limited and Christie Associates (1994) make no specific comment.

2 Royal College of Physicians (1994)

6.24 The College is conscious that differences of opinion on what should and what need not be subject to formal ethical review may pose difficulties for RECs; but it is of the nature of ethics that such differences occur, and achieving consensus can be difficult.

Non-medical research in human subjects

6.25 Naturally, it is in medical research that this College has most expertise and its primarily medical standpoint will be evident in much of the detail of this document: the general principles of ethical review have a wider application. The College believes that authorities which appoint RECs serving non-medical sciences will profit from this guide to ethical review of medical research. They will adapt the membership of any committee they appoint according to the kinds of studies to be reviewed.

Therapeutic trials

Design

6.26 Where two treatments are to be compared, it is often decided to allocate them at random, and, in order to obtain unbiased recording of the patient's progress, to conduct the study 'blind'. Where a placebo (or dummy medicine) is to be used as a control device in place of effective treatment, then the ethical issues require special consideration (see below).

6.27 When a new treatment or medication is investigated, its safety and efficacy are usually compared either with no treatment or with the best available or standard treatment.

Placebo

6.28 Treatment with placebo is a 'dummy' treatment or medication and participants are unaware whether they are receiving the active or placebo treatment; this is described as a 'blind' or 'masked' study. In order to obtain unbiased observation of the clinical results it is common practice that, where possible, the clinician also is unaware which of the treatments is active so that the experiment is then 'double blind'. The treatment groups may be formed by randomly allocating participants to separate groups or by giving each patient one or more periods of both active and placebo treatments in a 'cross-over' design. For conditions for which no effective treatment is known, placebo treatment groups do not present ethical problems, but where the placebo is used even temporarily instead of treatment believed to be effective, the issues require careful consideration of the patients' best interest which may include obtaining expert opinion as to the efficacy of that treatment.

6.29 The Declaration of Helsinki[1] refers to medical research combined with professional care, but does not, in theory, allow for controlled clinical trials in which there is a placebo arm unless there is no treatment of value. Placebo-controlled trials and other trials where there is no therapeutic intention, should be examined very critically if there is any possibility that they carry more than minimal risk. Licensing authorities such as the MCA or the US Food and Drugs Administration (FDA) often require comparisons with placebo, eg in the treatment of mild depression.

---

1 World Medical Association (1989)

6.30 Consent can often be obtained to the use of a placebo without impairing the scientific validity of the procedure: the patient is invited to agree that an inert preparation will (or may) be used and told why it will be used at some time during the course of treatment, but without specifying exactly when. The way in which the proposal is put to patients will vary with circumstances; the REC should satisfy itself that it will be done in such a way that patients can understand clearly what is implied without invalidating the experiment.

Withholding effective treatment

6.31 Withholding effective treatment for a short time, whether or not it is replaced by a placebo, can sometimes be acceptable in order to validate a technique of measurement or confirm the sensitivity of a therapeutic trial design. An investigator who proposes to do this should explicitly justify the intention, including consent procedure, and explain how it can be done without significant harm to the patient.

6.32 To choose a patient's medication, or to alter, shorten or prolong it, for the purpose of increasing enrolment in a study, is unethical.

Excluding high risk participants

6.33 In therapeutic trials, particularly those performed for the licensing of new medicines, it is common practice to exclude high risk participants. In one sense this is ethical in that it would be unethical to include participants who would be at materially greater than ordinary risk for any procedure. Thus, for example, it is proper to exclude pregnant women from early trials on the basis that their fetus is at unknown risk, until the benefits have been shown in non-pregnant individuals.

6.34 Some have argued, however, that this reduces the chance of such individuals benefiting in therapeutic research. In particular, it has been suggested that patients should not be excluded from trials from which they might benefit purely because they are elderly[1] or terminally ill. We suggest that exclusion of high risk individuals in the early stage of drug development should only be on the basis of risk to themselves or their offspring and not for administrative convenience or simply to protect commercial sponsors. Both the USA National Institutes of Health (NIH) and the FDA have recognised the need to ensure that women are adequately represented in clinical trials.[2,3]

6.35 CIOMS/WHO guidelines state that pregnant or nursing women should in no circumstances be the subjects of non-therapeutic research that carries more than minimal risk to the fetus or neonate, unless this is intended to elucidate problems of pregnancy or lactation.[4] These guidelines also state that as a general rule therapeutic research should be undertaken in pregnant or nursing women only with a view to improving the health of the mother without prejudice to that of the fetus or nursling, to enhancing the viability of the fetus, or to aiding the nursling's healthy development or the ability of the mother to nourish it adequately.

1 MRC (1994)

2 Bennet J C (1993)

3 Merkatz R B, Temple R, Sobel S, Feiden K and Kessler D A (1993)

4 CIOMS and WHO (1989)

6.36 This College considers that there can be legitimate research directed at benefiting the mother in which the possibility of fetal loss cannot be excluded.[1]

6.37 The possibility of an effect on the fetus should be addressed in the patient information sheet in all research involving pregnant women and RECs will closely scrutinise such proposals.

Informing general practitioners or other medical carers

6.38 A researcher must inform others who may be responsible for the medical care of patients or healthy volunteers of their participation in a trial. This will almost always require the researcher to notify the general practitioner when the patient is enrolled, with information about the possible medical implications of that involvement.

Informing participants after the research

6.39 Participation in research for the benefit of others should be acknowledged by the researcher by telling the participant about the results of the research where this is appropriate, of interest and practicable.

6.40 At the end of the study it may be appropriate to give participants some information about their personal involvement, such as revealing whether or not they received the placebo medication. This will be particularly necessary when the subject has, with the consent of the ethics committee, received only incomplete information because to tell all would have compromised the experiment (see 7.26).

1 British Paediatric Association and Royal College of Obstetricians and Gynacologists (1991)

7 ETHICAL ISSUES ARISING IN THE CONSIDERATION OF PROTOCOLS

Benefit and risk

7.1 As mentioned above, (see 1.10–1.11) there is a clear obligation on ethics committees to consider the balance of benefit and risk.

Risk

7.2 An excellent discussion of risk is given by Nicholson[1] and the reader is recommended to consult this work. In the USA and in the CIOMS/WHO guidelines, risk is classified as minimal, low (or minor increase over minimal) or high (greater than minor increase over minimal). Minimal risk could include everyday risks such as travelling on public transport or a private car (the latter having a considerably higher risk) but would not include travel by pedal or motorcycle; in medicine, they would be no more likely and not greater than the risk attached to routine medical or psychological examination.[2] Useful tables of various everyday, vocational and sporting risks are given by Nicholson. Minimal risk is where the chance of serious injury or death is very remote and may be ignored. Minimal risk may also be used for the situation where the level of distress or clinical malaise is slight or where there may be a chance of a reaction which is itself trivial, eg a mild headache, a feeling of lethargy or a dry mouth. Attempts have been made to quantify minimal risk as a risk of death of <1 per million or of major adverse effect of <10 per million, and low risk as 1 to 100 per million for death, and 10 to 1,000 per million for major adverse event.[3]

Benefit

7.3 Benefit may be weighed against risk in two different ways. First and most obviously, the patient may benefit. This is typified in a therapeutic trial where at least one of the treatments offered may be beneficial to the patient. Benefits may be considerable, for example, in cancer treatment and may counter balance even high risk to the individual. Second, society rather than the individual may benefit. In such situations, however large the benefit, to expose a participant to anything more than minimal risk needs very careful consideration and would rarely be ethical.

7.4 Note that benefit in this context is quite unrelated to any financial or other material benefit that the patient might receive as a result of participation. Such 'benefits' must be weighed with extreme care against risk. There is a general belief that in the past such 'benefits' may have been used inappropriately to encourage some dependent individuals (see 7.12–7.13) to participate in research studies.

Recruitment of healthy (non-patient) volunteers and patient volunteers

7.5 Consent should be sought of both healthy individuals and of patients.

1 Nicholson R H (1986)

2 CIOMS and WHO (1993), page 21

3 Nicholson R H (1986)

7.6 The College has produced reports on *Research on healthy volunteers*[1] and on *Research involving patients.*[2]

7.7 The view has been expressed that patients are not to be considered as volunteers, especially in therapeutic trials, because they are in a special position: they are ill, with the natural hope of getting better; they are dependent on the doctor; their understanding may be limited. But these factors are not so fundamental that they remove the voluntary element from participation. Patients who consent to enter a research study from which they may or may not benefit should be regarded as volunteers. Confusion would be avoided if the terms 'healthy (or non-patient) volunteer' and 'patient volunteer' were used. These factors make it particularly important to be scrupulous in obtaining consent. Investigators, particularly in non-therapeutic research, should realise that rather than the patients seeking help from the doctor, the doctor is now seeking help from them in the pursuit of new knowledge. It is suggested that the leading verb in letters to prospective participants should be 'invite'.

Payments to subjects

7.8 There is a tradition that healthy volunteer subjects should engage in research for purely idealistic or educational motives. Today, healthy volunteers cannot always be expected to participate in research without reward. Many investigations, eg studies of drug absorption and elimination, are tedious and time-consuming yet are done routinely, for example in the preparation of applications for licensing of medicines.

7.9 RECs should be informed of all proposed payments and should be satisfied that they are reasonable and not so large as to induce subjects to take risks which they would not otherwise take, nor to volunteer against their better judgement or more frequently than is advisable for their own good.[1] This applies to volunteer patients who may undertake extra activities or attendances which are therapeutically unnecessary as well as to healthy volunteers. Payments to patients should be especially closely scrutinised by RECs.

7.10 Agreements with volunteers to make themselves available on a panel basis to participate in a number of studies[3] (many of which may not be yet known or devised) require special scrutiny.

7.11 Reimbursement of subjects' expenses, eg for journeys, is not payment in the sense of reward; it is plainly desirable and should not be omitted. It has been suggested that acceptance of reimbursement or payment impairs the rights (ethical or legal) of subjects, but this is not so.

Dependent relationships

7.12 Subjects, both patient and non-patient, may be in a dependent relationship with investigators. Recruiting non-patient subjects, eg students, junior medical staff, nurses, employees of a pharmaceutical or other industry and members of the armed services, requires special care, including in some cases advice from an occupational

---

1 Royal College of Physicians (1986a)
2 Royal College of Physicians (1990)
3 Dudley H A F (1994)

physician. Calling for volunteers in institutions is best done in group situations, or by notices, rather than by direct individual approach.

7.13 The College reports on *Research on healthy volunteers*[1] and on *Research involving patients*[2] and the ABPI guidelines.[3] include advice on recruitment and selection, on special groups, (including children competent and non-competent to give consent, on people who are: elderly, terminally ill, members of ethnic minorities, suffering from a mental illness or with learning disability, prisoners, students or junior colleagues.

Institutions

7.14 If healthy volunteers are to be recruited in an institution, eg students or staff, then a responsible officer of that institution (eg dean, director of nurse education, works medical officer, personnel director) should be approached and general approval sought for recruitment to the project in case participation could adversely affect work performance or the welfare of the research subjects.

7.15 Many institutions have issued advice to students that they should satisfy themselves that any project they engage in has been approved by an independent ethics committee and that commercially sponsored projects should include a contract providing for the acceptance of liability for injury without regard to fault (see 9.26).

Developing communities

7.16 The CIOMS/WHO guidelines specifically address the issue of research with subjects in developing communities where special considerations are necessary, although these will not often concern LRECs in the United Kingdom.

Advertisements

7.17 Advertisements seeking volunteers, patient or non-patient, should be seen and approved by the REC or its representative in the institution in which they are to be published. Such advertisements should be restrained in tone and should not overstress payment or use the committee's approval as an inducement.

Knowledge of involvement and participant information

7.18 Subjects should always be made aware that they are involved in research, although to ensure this can sometimes be difficult or even impossible, eg in community projects or with children or people suffering from mental disability, or in medical emergencies (see Chapter 8).

7.19 The obvious impracticability of giving full information has led to the saying 'there is no such thing as informed consent', a criticism which is most easily rebutted by stressing that it is *adequate* or *sufficient* information that is required. The difficulties of what counts as adequate information are recognised in the various ways used to obtain consent (see 7.41–7.45).

7.20 In randomised trials patients should be told that a trial is in progress, that they will, if they consent to participate, be given either the standard treatment or one

---

1 Royal College of Physicians (1986a)

2 Royal College of Physicians (1990)

3 ABPI (1990)

which may prove to be better or worse, and that their treatment will be chosen by chance (random allocation). It has been suggested that patients may be allowed to express a preference for one or other treatment, including in the main analysis only those who give no preference.[1] This simply amounts to collecting information about a further group of patients who are not randomised, but it may improve recruitment.

7.21 Investigators are responsible for adequately counselling research subjects by word of mouth and by written material approved by the REC. But there are areas of particular complexity and sensitivity, such as research in human reproduction, where it may sometimes be appropriate to appoint a special informed person to act as independent counsellor to the subject. The investigator or the committee may propose this.

Withholding information from participants

7.22 Only in exceptional circumstances is there an argument for not telling patients that they are participating in research, for instance, when it would cause more distress to reveal the nature of the investigation and yet it is in the clinical interest of the patient to participate, or in some emergency medicine, or where the patient cannot understand. Acceptance of such an argument should be a deliberate decision taken as part of the ethical review (see 1.13). Discretionary practice of this sort would deflect the criticism that to obtain consent might be needlessly cruel.[2]

7.23 Where it is proposed to withhold from subjects information that would be material to a decision to participate, this should always be justified to an REC.

7.24 Where it is the investigator's medical opinion that disclosure of the information that would be adequate for consent would be so *harmful* that it would be unjustifiable, this can only be a decision about *individual* patients and only in therapeutic research and if the option is approved by the REC.

7.25 Approval to withhold information from all subjects in a study can be justified only in the most exceptional circumstances.

7.26 In some research the results may be compromised if the patient is given full information about the trial. For example, patients may not be given information which would allow them to discern which was active and which placebo treatment. Such 'deceptions' are good scientific practice and do not raise major ethical issues.

Deception

7.27 The need for ethically significant deception arises only very occasionally in biomedical research but may be more frequently necessary in psychological research as part of the experimental design. CIOMS/WHO guidelines state that deception is not permissible in research projects that carry more than minimal risk of harm to the subject. Furthermore, when deception is indispensable to the method of an experiment, the investigator must convince the REC first, that the experiment offers the acquisition of significant new knowledge, second, that no other research method would provide the answer, and third, that the deception would not inappropriately

1 Silverman W A (1994)

2 Tobias J S and Souhami R L (1993)

encourage participation of a reasonable person. It should be standard practice, after the experiment, to explain to subjects the reason for the deception.[1]

Written information sheets

7.28 Most research procedures should be the subject of an *information sheet* written in simple, easily comprehensible language. It should set out the purpose of the investigation, the procedures, the risks (including distress), the benefits or their absence to the individual or to other or future individuals or to society, a statement that the subjects may decline to participate (without incurring displeasure or any sort of penalty in the case of a dependent relationship, eg patient, student, employee), or withdraw at any time without giving a reason and without in any way impairing their care, and an invitation to ask questions. A statement about the arrangements and availability (or non-availability) of compensation for injury should be included wherever there is risk of physical injury (see 9.26). Approval by an REC or grant of a certificate by the medicines Licensing Authority (MCA) should not be referred to in a way that may cause potential volunteers to think that the project is specially recommended or is specially safe.

7.29 The information sheet for the patient or healthy volunteer is an important part of the process of seeking consent. It should always form part of the application to the REC.

7.30 Information sheets should clearly state the name, address and telephone number of the investigator and, if appropriate, of the person supervising the research.

Consent

Meaning of 'consent'

7.31 Potential research subjects are entitled to choose whether or not they will participate in research: obtaining valid (informed,* understanding, voluntary) consent is central to the ethical conduct of clinical investigation.

7.32 The terms 'valid', 'informed' and 'voluntary' imply that subjects have enough comprehensible information to enable them to make an uncoerced, deliberate (proper) judgement whether or not to participate. The word 'consent' encompasses these requirements, for if they are not met there is no true consent. In this document 'consent' is taken to mean informed and voluntary consent.

7.33 RECs should exercise discretion as to the mode of consent that is appropriate to the nature of the proposed research and the participants involved.

Impaired capacity

7.34 Where capacity to give consent is underdeveloped or impaired, for example in some individuals who are children, suffering from learning disability or mental illness or acutely ill and in some community/epidemiological research, special consideration is required (see 8.2–8.23).

---

* The term 'informed consent' carries specific legal meaning in the USA but not in the UK

1 British Psychological Society (1990)

7.35 An REC may agree that some research activities may be carried out without consent of the subject: some examples are listed in the 'Special classes of research' section (see Chapter 8).

Minor procedures

7.36 Minor procedures are those that have minimal risk (see 7.2) and entail no, or negligible, discomfort to a patient; in some instances to ask for formal consent would be more likely to cause distress to the patient than to proceed without it. In such cases, the criterion has been proposed that the procedures should not cause appreciably more discomfort than would be experienced by a patient undergoing routine diagnostic procedures for patient care, eg collection of urine and faeces, nasal and throat swabs and the withdrawal of a small extra volume of blood while blood is being taken for a necessary diagnostic process.

Major procedures

7.37 Major procedures which involve the subject in low or high risk can only be justified where considerable potential benefit exists. In some it may be impossible or devastating to obtain consent, for example, in unconscious patients, acute grave illness or inability to comprehend. In all cases, an REC will give close consideration to any proposal to proceed without consent of the subject or agreement of close relatives or friends, and will satisfy itself that the decision not to seek consent is ethically acceptable (see 8.18).

Refusal to participate and right to withdraw

7.38 Any fears of subjects that refusal to participate or decision to withdraw may lead to adverse consequences for themselves must be allayed. They must be assured that either decision will be accepted without question and that they will be treated as if the matter had not arisen.

Current conventional practice

7.39 There is no single preferred method of obtaining and recording consent that is appropriate to all research, but RECs should decide whether sufficient information has been provided, especially about potential risks and discomforts as well as any hoped for benefits, for an adequately informed choice to be possible.

7.40 It has often been suggested that where a randomised controlled trial is undertaken to compare conventional treatment with a novel treatment, then consent need formally be sought only from patients to whom the new treatment is allocated.[1] This technique (post-randomisation consent) involves withholding information on treatment options from patients and is usually unacceptable for that reason.

Modes of consent

Written or oral consent

7.41 Healthy volunteers and patient volunteers engaging in non-therapeutic research should give written consent to all but the most trivial procedures, such as measuring height and weight, or a single venepuncture in an adult. These minor procedures may be done with a simple explanation (set out in the application to the REC) and an oral response. In therapeutic research, consent procedures should be adapted to the circumstances of each case.

Written consent

7.42 Written consent has two protective functions, for subjects (who are in no doubt that they are entering research), and for investigators (where evidence of written consent may render them less vulnerable to litigation).

---

1 Lancet (1992)

7.43 There are various opinions on the value of written evidence of consent in the event of a legal action arising out of a clinical investigation. The likelihood is that a court of law would look at any such document in the context of the whole investigation and might at best regard it as evidence that the investigator has seriously endeavoured to meet responsibilities, and at worst dismiss it as meaningless or misleading. A written consent in no way reduces the responsibilities of an investigator and of itself does not remove the ordinary rights of the subject. It can be withdrawn by the subject orally and at any time.

Consent form

7.44 The subjects should be given plenty of time to study the information sheet, to consult their families or their general practitioners where appropriate, and may then sign a form that states that the information sheet has been studied and discussed with the investigator and that the subject agrees to participate. This is probably less intimidating than a single large consent form incorporating all the information. A standard hospital 'Consent to Treatment' form is not appropriate to research.

Witnessed consent

7.45 Witnessed consent is especially useful for those who have intellectual or cultural difficulties in speech or understanding, or who are distressed but deemed capable of giving consent. An independent person signs a document stating that the witness was present when the investigator explained the project to the potential subject and that in the witness's opinion consent was given freely and with understanding.

7.46 Where *incapacity to consent is transient*, explanation to the subject, when he or she is able to receive it, is desirable (see 8.18).

Retention of documents

7.47 Copies of consent documents should be kept in the subject's case records (where these exist) for the statutory life of the record, as well as in research records for 15 years.

Developments in consent procedures in patients

7.48 Developments in consent procedures in patients are taking place and it is appropriate to consider one source of concern about current practice. Some people are averse to asking patients to sign a statement indicating that they consent to participate in a study because they believe this can be misleading and even intimidating. A signed consent form, in the event of a dispute between investigator and patient, might be used to protect the investigator rather than the patient. This creates a conflict of interests which is avoided by appropriate wording of consent and information sheets.

7.49 As an alternative to seeking consent forms signed by patients, it has been suggested that it may be better to be able to demonstrate consent by keeping suitably detailed records of the consultation (see 7.45–7.46) and, where appropriate, by having given the patient written information and the opportunity to think further before making a decision. In most circumstances, however, seeking a signature from patients may help to emphasise that what is proposed is research rather than standard practice; it may be thought appropriate to invite patients to sign a simple statement that they have received detailed information on the study rather than a consent form.

Questionnaires

7.50 Questionnaires, copies of which should be supplied to the REC, are often innocuous and may even be offered by mail. The fact that the subject completes the questionnaire can be taken as consent, provided that the letter of invitation expressly leaves the subject free of obligation.

7.51 Some investigations may involve questionnaires that are intrusive and may cause distress or resentment if presented to the subject without preparation. For such questionnaires it is appropriate to seek the subject's consent before the questionnaire is offered.

7.52 RECs should be flexible about consent procedures regarding questionnaires.

The use of video/audio recordings

8.1 Audio or video recordings present special problems, particularly in relation to consent.[1,2] At the time of agreeing to participate the subject will not know the content of the recording. It is common and good practice to ask for additional consent after the recording has been made and offer the opportunity to review the recording if they wish. The consent should include a specific description of the uses (eg for teaching) that will be made of the material, and the audience or research staff to whom it will become available. The participant should be assured in advance that withdrawal of consent after the recording will result in erasure of the material. Ethics committees need to be assured that secondary loan or copying will not be a cause of the material being used for other than the agreed purposes and audiences.

Vulnerable participants

Research involving children

8.2 The particular problems relating to research involving children have been the subject of several reports and a book.[3] The British Paediatric Association (BPA) published revised guidelines in 1992[4] and has a Standing Ethics Advisory Committee which will respond to requests for advice but not for approval of protocols from individuals or from ethics committees.

8.3 It may well be appropriate to give medical treatment to unwilling children if the parent or guardian consents, but the position would not necessarily be the same for research. In legal terms (in England and Wales) a person is of full age, and accordingly recognised as an adult, from the eighteenth birthday. Under that age, the capacity to consent to research depends on the degree of understanding on the part of the individual concerned. The Family Law Reform Act 1969 states that the consent of a person between 16 and 18 years of age to surgical, medical or dental treatment shall be as effective as it would be if the patient were of full age, so that parental consent is not necessary. 'Treatment' includes diagnostic and ancillary procedures, including the administration of an anaesthetic, and thus probably includes therapeutic research, but it would not be prudent to rely solely on the subject's consent to non-therapeutic research, and below the age of 18 parental consent should always be sought in addition to that of the subject. In Scotland the position in law is slightly different: valid consent may be given by girls older than 12 and boys older than 14 rather than the 16 year demarcation in England and Wales.[5]

8.4 To the extent that is feasible, which will vary with age, the willing co-operation of the child should be sought, after he or she has been frankly informed of any possible discomfort or inconvenience. Older children may be assumed to be capable

1 Royal College of General Practitioners (1993)

2 GMC (1995)

3 Nicholson R H (1989)

4 British Paediatric Association (1992)

5 MRC (1991b)

of giving consent preferably also with the consent of the parent or other legal guardian. Where a child obviously objects to such research, ie he or she withholds assent or agreement, or resists, this must be respected.

8.5 There must be no financial or other inducement to parent, guardian or child.[1] Children should not be the subject of research that might equally well be carried out on adults. However, their participation is indispensable for research on diseases of childhood and conditions to which children are particularly susceptible.

8.6 A semantic problem has arisen over the question as to whether venepuncture carries a greater than 'minimal' risk in children. The BPA guidelines should be read in conjunction with the commentary by the president of the BPA included as an addendum in later editions. We do not consider venepuncture to have more than a minimal risk in normal circumstances.

8.7 Children should in no circumstances be the subjects of research holding no potential benefit for them unless with the objective of elucidating physiological or pathological conditions peculiar to infancy and childhood, or of providing potential benefit to the family, and where it involves no more than minimal risk.

Pregnant and nursing women

8.8 The CIOMS/WHO guidelines[2] advise that no special problems of eliciting consent exist in the case of pregnant and nursing mothers as such, though many committees require that consent to research is not sought in the immediate period around childbirth unless this is unavoidable.

People who suffer from mental illness or learning disability

8.9 Substantially similar ethical considerations apply to people who suffer from mental illness or learning disability as apply to children. They should never be the subjects of research that might equally well be carried out in adults in full health, but they are clearly the only subjects available for some research into the origins and treatment of mental disease or disability.

8.10 Many people who suffer from mental illness or learning disability are competent to understand the implications of research and to make up their own minds whether they wish to take part.

8.11 Difficult questions arise where competence is in doubt or is clearly impaired.

8.12 A significant difference between those suffering mental illness as opposed to learning disability that should be taken into account is that incompetence may be transient in the case of the former. See also the College Report on *Research involving patients*[3] and guidelines on psychiatric research.[4]

8.13 Again there are differences in the law between that in England and Wales, in Scotland and in the European Union.[5] A law commission report gives an interpreta-

---

1 Royal College of Physicians (1990)

2 CIOMS and WHO (1993)

3 Royal College of Physicians (1990)

4 Royal College of Psychiatrists (1989)

5 MRC (1991c)

tion of the law relating to medical interventions in people suffering from mental incapacity.[1]

8.14 In the UK where an adult suffering from physical or mental illness or learning disability is not competent to give consent, there is no provision in law for another individual to give consent on his or her behalf.

8.15 The CIOMS/WHO Guidelines[2] also state:

> 'The agreement of the immediate family, whether spouse, parent, adult offspring or sibling, should be sought but is sometimes of doubtful value, especially as families sometimes regard persons with mental or behavioural disorders as an unwelcome burden. In the case of a person who has been committed to an institution by a court order, it may be necessary to seek legal authorisation for involving the person in research.'

Therapeutic research

8.16 A recent decision of the House of Lords, made in a case of *treatment* of a mentally handicapped person, establishes that a doctor may proceed without consent, provided the action is in the best interest of the patient and in accordance with a practice accepted by a responsible body of medical opinion.[3] The relatives should be consulted. The court was not concerned with *research*, but these principles might apply to therapeutic research which involves treatment chosen for a patient in the exercise of the investigator's clinical judgement.

Non-therapeutic research

8.17 A strong ethical case for non-therapeutic research can be made where that research involves no more than minimal risk; progress in treatment is dependent on better understanding of mental illness and learning disability. We consider that the best guidance for such research might be that there should be agreement by the close relatives or guardians and that the patient seems to agree to the procedure. No patient who refuses or, if incapable of refusing, resists should be included in, or continue in, research. Where no relative is available or, as sometimes happens, a patient desires privacy and does not wish relatives to be informed, another designated person, approved by the LREC, should be consulted.[4]

Unconscious or acutely ill patients

8.18 The problems are similar to those described above but in some cases, eg treatment of acute cardiac emergencies, the question arises of what, if anything, the patient or family should be told later. The LREC should advise on this. Informing patients that they are participants in a trial after entry, even if offering the possibility of withdrawal, may not prevent their inclusion as contributors to the data in an 'intention to treat' design.[5] This does not appear to be a major ethical issue while the right to withdraw from active involvement clearly is.

---

1 Law Commission (1995)

2 CIOMS and WHO (1993)

3 West Berkshire Health Authority (1989)

4 Royal College of Physicians (1990)

5 Hall A S (1994)

Other vulnerable groups

8.19 The quality of the consent of candidate subjects who are junior or subordinate members of a hierarchically-structured group or are prisoners requires careful consideration. Willingness to volunteer may be unduly influenced by the expectation, whether justified or not, of adventitious benefits.

Community-based research

8.20 Some community research is so unintrusive that individual consent is not necessary. The principles of confidentiality should be preserved

8.21 The CIOMS/WHO guidelines conclude that:

> 'Where research is undertaken on a community basis for example by experimental treatment of water supplies, by health services research or by large-scale trials of new insecticides, of new prophylactic or immunising agents, and of nutritional adjuvants or substitutes individual consent on a person-to-person basis may not be feasible, and the ultimate decision to undertake the research will rest with the responsible public health authority in consultation with an REC. The committee should satisfy itself that it is permissible to proceed without individual consent and that the investigator or sponsor has made adequate arrangements to protect the safety of the research subjects and maintain confidentiality, eg by anonymous reporting of results.'

8.22 These guidelines[1] also state that all possible means should be used to inform the community concerned of the aims of the research, the advantages expected from it, and any possible hazards or inconveniences. If feasible, dissenting individuals should have the option of withholding their participation. Whatever the circumstances, the ethical considerations and safeguards applied to research on individuals must be translated, in every possible respect, into the community context.

8.23 CIOMS and WHO have published separate guidelines for epidemiological research.[2]

Unintrusive research

Anonymous data and personal medical records

8.24 There is a duty to use available information for the general good where this can be done without detriment. Use of identifiable personal data or materials without approaching or involving the patients concerned is, in principle, ethically acceptable on the same basis as community research (above) provided that confidentiality is preserved or the data are anonymous and that the individual concerned has not opted out of anonymous testing.*

8.25 Where anonymity of data cannot be reversed it has been considered that individual consent is neither necessary nor appropriate (eg HIV prevalence in pregnant women)

---

* There is a provision for example for individuals to give notice that they wish to opt out of anonymous HIV testing.

1 CIOMS and WHO (1993)

2 CIOMS and WHO (1991)

8.26 Even when data are not anonymous but confidentiality is assured, RECs may feel it reasonable not to ask individuals for their consent to the use of their personal medical records, register-held information or existing biological samples for research purposes.

8.27 Where patients who have a particular condition are identified by scanning registers and it is desired to approach them with a view to research, this should be done through their family doctor or consultant.

Use of discarded tissues for research

8.28 The use for research of anonymous tissues genuinely discarded in the course of medical treatment, for example, discarded blood samples, pleural fluid, or leftover biopsy tissue, and of tissues removed at surgery or at autopsy, is a traditional and ethically acceptable practice, that we suggest does not need consent from patients or relatives and may not need to be submitted to an REC (see Appendix B). There may be legal constraints and it remains unclear to whom such samples belong in terms of beneficial ownership. Commercial exploitation of a protein from such a sample has, in the USA, resulted in a claim for profit-sharing by the patient.[1] The research and therapeutic uses of human tissue have been the subject of a report by the Nuffield Council of Bioethics.[2] Fetal tissue (see below) is subject to special guidelines.

8.29 Hospitals or health authorities may be approached by companies interested in purchasing human materials, eg pleural fluid, protein from which can be useful in diagnostic assays. RECs may reasonably respond to a request to advise on the ethical conduct of such sales in this borderline area of research and medical practice. Patient consent need not be sought. Money received should pass to the health authority and there should be no personal gain to the staff involved (except as salary from their employer).

Fetuses and fetal material

8.30 The *Review of the guidance on the research use of fetuses and fetal material* (the Polkinghorne Report) was published in July 1989[3] and the DoH has published guidance based on this.[4] The College supports the view of the Polkinghorne Committee that a Code of Practice that is accepted and implemented by the profession allows necessary flexibility and is preferable to legislation. All RECs should have copies of the Polkinghorne Report available for consultation whenever the use of fetuses or fetal material is proposed.

8.31 Item 6 of the Code of Practice proposed by the Polkinghorne Committee states:

> 'All research, or therapy of an innovative character, involving the fetus or fetal tissue should be described in a protocol and be examined by an ethics committee. Projects should be subject to review until the validity of the procedure has been recognised by the committee as part of routine medical practice. The ethics committee has a duty to examine the progress of the research or innova-

1 Moore v Regents of the University of California.

2 Nuffield Council of Bioethics (1995)

3 Polkinghorne (1989)

4 Department of Health (1995)

tive therapy (eg by receiving reports). It should have access to records and be able to confirm that the material is in fact being used for the purpose set out in the protocol. It should also be able to examine the record of any financial transactions involving fetal tissue. Before permitting research the ethics committee must satisfy itself:

a of the validity of the research or use proposed;

b that the objectives of the proposed use cannot be achieved in any other way;

c that the researchers or clinicians have the necessary facilities and skill.'

In vitro fertilisation and embryos

8.32 In this particularly sensitive area of medical practice the Polkinghorne committee recommended that protocols for treatment as well as research were submitted to research ethics committees (see above). It is no longer necessary to submit protocols when a treatment licence has been granted by the HFEA (see also A1.15–A1.16).

8.33 For research protocols relating to *in vitro* fertilisation and other methods of assisted reproduction, gene, embryo, fetal and transplant research — RECs should refer to the guidelines issued by the HFEA, GTAC or other authorities where applicable and, when there is a need for specialist opinion not already available within the committee, consult or co-opt (see 4.9).

8.34 The guidelines of the HFEA and of the Polkinghorne Committee agree that no request for the use of abortion fetal material may be made until after the decision to terminate pregnancy has been taken. They differ, however, in that the HFEA would allow the mother to specify whether the aborted material may be put to research or to therapeutic use, whereas the Polkinghorne Committee would not. RECs must decide which recommendation to follow in cases where the HFEA has no jurisdiction. They may feel that, granted that all the safeguards against pressure are in place, consent to specified use is, in principle, the more desirable option.

Gene therapy

8.35 As with embryo research, the government set up a committee (The Clothier Committee) to examine and report on the ethics of these novel scientific interventions. The Gene Therapy Advisory Committee is established on a non-statutory basis to consider applications of gene therapy and to keep developments under review. It has published guidelines for applicants with useful appendices.[1] It does not supplant the work of RECs.

HIV/AIDS

8.36 The advent of HIV/AIDS has raised a number of apparently novel ethical issues in research and practice. The question of anonymous testing without consent is covered elsewhere (see 8.24–8.29) and the MRC has published guidelines for conduct of AIDS vaccine trials.[2]

---

1 Gene Therapy Advisory Committee (1994)

2 MRC (1991d)

9 INJURIES DURING CLINICAL RESEARCH

The legal position

9.1 If an accident occurs, the present legal position is that the individual (patient or healthy volunteer) who is injured is entitled to compensation if negligence on the part of the research worker or the team or a supplier of drugs or equipment can be shown (fault liability) or if it can be shown that the 'producer' has supplied a 'defective' product (strict liability under the Consumer Protection Act 1987). Since one of the purposes of medical research is to explore the unknown and to discover if there are any unforeseen or unforeseeable consequences of what is being investigated, accidents may occur despite the greatest care.

Ex gratia payments

9.2 When an injury occurs, another means by which a participant or dependant might receive some compensation, whether or not negligence is alleged, would be by seeking an *ex gratia* * payment from the sponsor of the research or the authority employing the researcher. The Consumer Protection Act 1987 reverses the burden of proof from the injured person to the manufacturer but is otherwise unlikely materially to alter the position in respect of research involving pharmaceutical products. This is because the manufacturer is allowed the 'development risk' or 'state of the art' defence, ie that the adverse effect was not predictable by currently known scientific tests. In addition, that a warning was given may also be taken into account in determining whether the product should be treated as 'defective' under the Act.

Compensation for injury

9.3 The situation regarding compensation for injury due to participation in research without legal proof of liability is currently unsatisfactory. Some issues will have to await solution on a national basis and there is little that individual RECs can do about them.

Healthy volunteers

9.4 Where research sponsored by an industrial company involves healthy volunteers or patients, clear guidelines exist and compensation is almost universally provided for.

9.5 The Association of the British Pharmaceutical Industry (ABPI) has published for its members guidelines on compensation for injury.[1] These are advisory only, and not all pharmaceutical companies are members of the Association. Contract research companies are not eligible for membership of the ABPI. The College considers that where medical research on healthy volunteers is undertaken by contract companies

---

* An *ex gratia* payment is one that is voluntarily made without admission that it is legally due.

1 ABPI (1991)

on behalf of a pharmaceutical company, it should be made clear whether the sponsor or contract company is responsible for compensation.[1]

9.6 In all studies in healthy volunteers sponsored by a pharmaceutical or other company, including those testing or sponsoring tests of industrial chemicals, cosmetics, instruments and appliances or devices, a contract which accepts liability regardless of fault should be used for each subject. A contract cannot be made without the agreement of both parties. The ABPI recommends a text for such a contract in its *Guidelines for medical experiments in non-patient human volunteers.*[2]

9.7 The ABPI *Draft provisions for volunteer agreement and consent form* are satisfactory insofar as they provide for compensation by the sponsoring company for injury caused directly by participation in the study without the subject having to prove either negligence or that the product was defective in the sense that it did not fulfil a reasonable expectation of safety. These guidelines and contracts are also appropriate for use by non-pharmaceutical companies testing industrial or household chemicals or pesticides.

9.8 The legal situation for subjects who participate in research funded by state bodies such as universities, health authorities or trusts, by research organisations such as the MRC, or originated by individual research workers, is much less satisfactory.

9.9 Many organisations and institutions already have third party liability policies that cover negligence. We recommend that policies be extended to cover compensation payable under such contracts independent of proof of negligence. The number of claims is likely to be small and the extra insurance premium should be acceptable.

9.10 In studies involving healthy volunteers the Medicines Commission has recommended that there should be an assurance in advance of adequate compensation without the need for the volunteer to show negligence.

9.11 Public sector bodies may have difficulty in implementing such a contract procedure, but the MRC has stated that it will give sympathetic consideration to making *ex gratia* payments.

9.12 It is important that the organisation or institution responsible for compensation be named in the protocol and the contract form, and that RECs ensure that this has been done. In the event of a dispute or difference of opinion regarding a claim including the issue of negligence by a third party, we advise following the procedure suggested by the ABPI:[2] that reference be made to an arbitrator or arbitrators appointed by the President of the appropriate medical Royal College, the arbitrator having the power to consult a barrister with regard to any issue of law including the amount of compensation.

Existing legal rights

9.13 As the law stands, if injury or ill health occurs as a result of failure to take care by the investigator or anyone else, the volunteer still has the alternative of pursuing a claim for negligence. The wording of the contract should be such that the volunteer

1 Royal College of Physicians (1986a)

2 ABPI (1990)

would not waive any existing legal rights against the organisation or institution or any person involved in the research.

Patients

9.14 The position regarding patients is inevitably more complex than with healthy volunteers, particularly with regard to acceptance of risk.

9.15 It is our view that the same general principles and arrangements should apply in clinical trials involving patients as those described above for healthy volunteer studies. The agreement with the patient, while based on an information sheet and consent form rather than a contract, should be equally clear both to the participant and the REC.

Industry sponsored investigations

9.16 The situation is straightforward for industry sponsored trials since the ABPI have published guidelines[1] which RECs should require sponsors to agree in writing to accept and apply.

9.17 Companies can be expected to pay compensation only if there is reasonable 'balance of probability' evidence of causation. The ABPI guidelines commit companies only to 'favourably consider' claims.

9.18 In the case of pre-marketing trials on patients of new medicines (or trials of marketed medicines for new, unlicensed, indications) sponsored by industrial companies, the ABPI recommends member companies to accept, 'without legal commitment', the responsibility for compensating patients for injury (with some exclusions). However, the ABPI has advised member companies that with the completion of the study the special arrangements should no longer apply in relation, for instance, to patients continuing treatment with an unlicensed medicine on a 'named-patient' basis (see A1.13). Also, these guidelines do not apply where a marketed medicine (having a Product Licence) is studied in further trials for its licensed indication. The guidelines exclude compensation for injury due to failure of clinical effect of either the medicine under investigations or during placebo treatments unless this was specifically agreed in the proposal, eg a contraceptive trial.

9.19 Companies may agree to delete the exclusion clauses relating to licensed medicines or placebo phases.

9.20 Where there are extra investigations that carry some risk (eg endoscopies), companies can reasonably be expected to accept responsibility for these as well as for the medicine itself and the ABPI guidelines recognise this by specifying injury caused by *participation* and not only due to the drug.

Non-industry sponsored investigations

9.21 It is not to be expected that pharmaceutical companies will accept responsibility on this basis for any study they have not sponsored or initiated.

9.22 Participants in research sponsored by non-industrial organisations (eg academic, charitable, state) which are not members of any trade association might

---

1 ABPI (1991)

reasonably expect to be offered compensation for injury on similar terms to those of the ABPI guidelines and European Community guidelines.[1,2]

9.23 Some state funded organisations (including DoH, HAs, NHS Trusts, Research Councils, etc) are not permitted by the government to make such 'open ended' agreements in advance nor to insure their risk. Some universities and public sector bodies are insured not only for legal liability but also for 'no fault compensation'.*

9.24 The MRC has stated it will give sympathetic consideration to making *ex gratia* payments. Other research organisations, eg the Higher Education Funding Council and the DoH have a similar policy, and such payments have in the past been made.

What an REC can do in practice

Responsibility

9.25 The LREC can point out the position regarding responsibility for injury to research subjects, to its appointing authority and to grant-giving bodies supporting research that is before it, and ask for a reply either in general terms or in respect of an individual project, and take their reply into consideration in its review.

Availability of compensation

9.26 The REC will recognise that it has not hitherto been the practice to advise all research subjects (patient and healthy) of the availability or non-availability of compensation for injury, that it would be irrelevant to do so in some cases (eg a questionnaire) and inappropriate to do so in others (eg some cancer trials where, for example, a treatment may carry a high, but acknowledged and accepted risk). Where the committee thinks that the risks of the investigation warrant it, such information should be provided in the information sheet. Research subjects who are accepting risk are entitled to the information that is material to their decision to participate and it is for the committee to judge when it is appropriate to inform subjects of their position in this regard. Subjects who are injured, and/or who feel they have been misled on this matter, eg on the availability of prompt compensation, may feel sufficiently aggrieved to accuse the committee of failing in its duty of care, and even to issue a writ for negligence (see 3.4–3.6).

Studies sponsored by industrial companies

9.27 Sponsorship is deemed to exist where a company initiates or supports a study. Companies, whether or not they are members of the ABPI, should accept in writing the current appropriate ABPI guidelines relating to compensation for injury to patients[3] or provide a written statement that delivers at least the same protection. For non-patient (healthy) volunteers ABPI guidelines[4] which provide for individual contracts should be implemented. Companies may have their own no fault compensation conditions that are more favourable to patients than the ABPI guidelines. In such

---

* No fault compensation insurance by Universities and Postgraduate Institutes. Personal Communication. Registrar of the RCP.

1 ABPI (1991)

2 EC (1991b)

3 ABPI (1991)

4 ABPI (1990)

cases committees may welcome such initiatives but be reassured by written confirmation that the company agrees to abide by ABPI guidelines (thus ensuring this level of protection as a minimum and avoiding the need for legal scrutiny of complex statements). Companies may also be persuaded to 'improve' the protection offered (See 9.19)

9.28 Some foreign companies and their UK-based subsidiaries have, in the past, objected to accepting ABPI compensation guidelines. The problem can normally be overcome by firm persistence.

Funds for compensation from industry sources

9.29 If a proper undertaking to compensate in accordance with applicable guidelines is given by a major company it is probably not appropriate for an REC to enquire whether it will be discharged out of company funds or the proceeds of an insurance policy; these are matters for the company to decide.

Non-industry sponsored research

Public sector bodies

9.30 Public sector and other bodies (university, MRC, DoH), who may have difficulty in implementing contract procedures for *healthy volunteers*, may be asked for an assurance that the *ex gratia* position would be implemented to give protection similar to that recommended by this College and adopted by the ABPI.

Insurance of research subjects

9.31 Recently, insurance companies have invited universities and other research organisations to take out insurance to cover injury to research subjects, whether or not the injury is due to negligence. At present most have legal liability insurance only (ie confined to negligence).

Indemnity to health authority

9.32 The issue arises as to what indemnity (if any) the person or organisation sponsoring research should give to the investigator, the relevant health authority or other institution whose facilities or staff are being used. Such indemnities relate to protecting investigators and employers rather than to protecting research subjects in the event that a claim arises. Such indemnities are not a necessary concern of RECs; they should be left to the parties to negotiate as they see fit. These indemnities often provide for the handling of any legal proceedings by the company. This would not seem to disadvantage research subjects.

9.33 Medical researchers will usually be either members of a medical protection organisation which will look after their interests or may be accorded indemnity by an employing health authority provided that the research is part of the employed investigator's duties. Investigators should check with employers regarding indemnity for research activity both for themselves and other staff involved, eg junior staff, nurses etc.

10 PAYMENTS TO RESEARCHERS

Investigators, departments and institutions

10.1 Any pecuniary relationship of an investigator to a sponsoring company has ethical implications and should be declared to the LREC giving details of both the amount and nature (money, gifts, travel etc), of payments to investigators. The same applies to payments to departments and to institutions by a pharmaceutical company or a contract research company.[1]

Declaration of interest

10.2 Personal or departmental involvement in a company or direct ownership of its shares (excepting ownership where decided by a fund manager) are interests that should be declared.

General Medical Council advice

10.3 The GMC provides examples of 'inducements which the Council may regard as improper':[2]

> *'Clinical trials of drugs'.* 'It is unethical for a doctor to accept per capita or other payments from a pharmaceutical firm in relation to a research project such as the clinical trial of a new drug, unless the payments have been specified in a protocol * for the project which has been approved by the relevant national or local ethical committee. It may be improper for a doctor to accept per capita or other payments under arrangements for recording clinical assessments of a licensed medicinal product, whereby he is asked to report reactions which he has observed in patients for whom he has prescribed the drug, unless the payments have been specified in a protocol for the project which has been approved by a relevant research ethics committee. It is improper for a doctor to accept payment in money or kind which could influence the professional assessment of the therapeutic value of a new drug, or of its appropriateness for a particular patient'.
>
> *'Gifts and loans'.* 'It may be improper for an individual doctor to accept from a pharmaceutical firm monetary gifts or loans of expensive items of equipment for personal use'.

Royal College of Physicians advice

10.4 Payments to researchers are also discussed in the RCP report on *The relationship between physicians and the pharmaceutical industry.*[1]

---

* Details of financial arrangements are often included in an investigator agreement, available to the LREC but separate from the main protocol for reasons of confidentiality.

1 Royal College of Physicians (1986b)

2 GMC (1987)

Recruitment of subjects for reward

10.5 The RCP recognises the conflict that exists between the need of the sponsor to have an agreement with the investigator that reflects the amount of work done and the view that *per capita* payments may tempt investigators inappropriately to recruit patients to studies or to retain them improperly when recruited. It is suggested that rewards to investigators should, as far as possible, not simply reflect numbers recruited and should not therefore be solely *per capita* based.

10.6 Doctors may be asked to recruit patients to a study in which they are not personally involved. Financial reward for such recruitment is unethical.

Role of the REC

10 7 RECs have a particular responsibility to examine closely all financial arrangements, particularly where there may be an element of inducement to recruit patients (see discussion in RCP report on *Research involving patients.*[1])

10.8 Rates of payment to investigators for participation in clinical trials should reflect actual work carried out (eg, time spent, staff employed, consumables, etc) with personnel costs reflecting normal rates* for the professional involved (eg doctor, nurse, secretary etc).

---

* The Clinical Research Ethics Committee of the RCGP suggests that BMA scales for GP private consultations are appropriate. We suggest that BUPA consultation rates for consultants would be a useful guideline. The BMA also publishes guidelines for fees for work for pharmaceutical companies, updated in its Fees Supplement. These have been endorsed by the ABPI.

1 Royal College of Physicians (1990)

11 APPLICATIONS TO THE ETHICS COMMITTEES

Nature of the application

11.1 RECs should deal directly with the investigators who bear responsibility for the subjects of the research, even though the protocol may have been provided by another, for example, a pharmaceutical company.

11.2 Applications that have been prepared by junior staff or others who do not bear ultimate clinical responsibility for the research subjects should, before they are sent to the committee, be scrutinised for the quality of both science and ethics by a senior or other person who does bear this responsibility, eg, an NHS consultant who agrees to research being done by others on patients under his or her care (see 1.14). This is no mere formality; the clinician's responsibility to patients includes research studies carried out with their consent.

Format

11.3 Research projects vary greatly. A standard format, though not always appropriate, can save much time since it ensures that applicants do not omit essential matter. *An example* of a format which committees can adopt or adapt to their own needs, follows at the end of this section. A very detailed format is given by Bendall.[1] Forms to be completed by applicants are in use by many LRECs and have been standardised with considerable benefit and general acceptability in at least two regions (Northern and South West).

Clarity of language

11.4 It should be stressed that applications must include at least a full summary of the project and the ethical issues raised in language that can be understood by *all* members of the committee. Nevertheless, a medical dictionary or other text[2] may be useful for each member.

11.5 With the formal or highly technical protocol, a brief summary in lay terms and plan of the research with an overview of the way in which subjects are to be involved and any risks to which they may be exposed, should be supplied. The patient (subject) information sheet may help a great deal in this regard.

Special considerations

11.6 It can be useful for the applicant to review the application with an independent experienced clinical scientist or statistician or with a scientific advisory group appointed by the main committee, where this is practicable. Such consultation allows the identification of obvious errors and inadequacies and promotes clear presentation to the RECs as well as reducing delay.

---

1 Bendall C (1994)

2 The Merck manual is one such useful text

11.7 The REC may also issue guidelines with the object of minimising difficulties and delays resulting from the excessive use of technical terminology, confusion over the regulatory status of a new drug, product liability, consent, data protection legislation etc. Copies of these guidelines and access to other material should be available to applicants.

11.8 For all studies on hospital inpatients, the approval of the consultant responsible for their overall care is required.

Consulting with colleagues

11.9 Investigators are responsible for consulting with colleagues and/or other groups who may be involved or affected by the research, for example, the consultant or general practitioner in charge of the overall care of the patient, with heads of laboratories to which samples may be sent, with pharmacists, nurses or community workers. The institution where the research is to be carried out will normally need reassurance that all additional costs to themselves are met from within the budget of the research or that these costs are agreed by them as an appropriate call on their budget. Note that all health authorities and trusts have obligations and contracts to support research.

11.10 *Nursing and other staff* should always be made aware that research in progress in patients with whom they are concerned has been approved by an REC.

11.11 *Hospital pharmacists* should know what drugs are being used in the institution, whether on inpatients or outpatients and will normally be involved in their supply: they should be told of drug studies whether or not they are involved in their supply.

Good clinical practice

11.12 Guidelines for good clinical [research] practice (GCP) were first published by ABPI in 1988 for the use of companies carrying out trials where the data were to be used for licence applications. The current edition[1] accords with EC directives and GCP guidelines.[2]

11.13 **Suggested checklist for information to be provided to RECs**

1 State the title of the proposed project.

2 State the name and post of the principal investigator and the site at which the research will take place. State the names and posts of all investigators involved.

3 State the name(s) of the person(s) carrying clinical responsibility for patients or research subjects.

4 State the question to be answered and the value of answering it.

5 State the name of the responsible permanent member of staff (eg consultant, head of department, etc) if the research is being carried out by a junior or temporary member of a department.

6 State the sponsorship for the study and the financial arrangements between sponsor and investigator for the research contract or agreement.

1 ABPI (1992)

2 EC (1990, 1991)

7 State the personal experience of the applicant in the field of investigation concerned.

8 Give an outline in straightforward language of the proposed project, including the procedures to be used, the measurements to be made and how the data will be analysed. The latter may include statements of method (eg intention to treat, statistical materials) and should include relevant information about the statistical power of the protocol.

9 If the project is designed to test a *drug or appliance* state its exact regulatory status (see Appendix A).

10 Specify the number of subjects, whether they are patients or other, who will be involved, how they will be recruited, whether they are in a dependent relationship with the investigator, eg student, or whether specially vulnerable, eg children, people suffering from learning disability or mental illness.

11 State inclusion and exclusion criteria for subjects. If in a special group, eg children, see Chapter 8 for a review of information required.

12 State the potential hazards to subjects, if any, their estimated probability (if possible) and the precautions to be taken to meet them. Radiation hazards require an appropriate certificate confirming that researchers have attended a course for persons clinically or physicially directing radiation exposure. (Housing Regulation 1988 Statutory Instrument No 778.)

13 State the procedures which may cause discomfort or distress to subjects and the degree of discomfort or distress entailed, and their estimated probability.

14 Provide a copy of the subject information sheet or state why none is needed.

15 State the manner in which the subject's consent will be obtained (if written, include a copy).

16 State whether the subject's general practitioner is to be informed of a patient's recruitment before the study begins, and whether the subject's consent to such information being passed on is a condition of participation.

17 Attach any other relevant matter: for instance, letters to subjects (which *must* be in simple, non-technical language), payments to subjects, copies of advertisements or any other recruiting matter for healthy or patient volunteers etc.

18 State the likely duration of the project and the premises in which it will be undertaken.

19 State what, if any, arrangements have been made for compensation in the event of injury to subjects (where there is neither fault nor liability under the Consumer Protection Act).

20 If the study is sponsored by an industrial company the specific arrangement including agreement to abide by ABPI guidelines (current edition 1991) should be specified.

21 State any 'interest', ie of profit, personal or departmental, financial or otherwise, relating to the study.

APPENDIX A

Development and official regulation of medicines
(Medicines Act 1968)

Phases of clinical trials of medicines and vaccines

A1.1 It is important for the REC to understand the phases of development of drugs and vaccines since different regulations apply and different types of participant may be involved.

A1.2 In **Phase I trials** new drugs are administered for the first time to humans and the participants are generally healthy volunteers. Phase I studies may, however, include patient volunteers — either where toxicity precludes administration to healthy volunteers (eg anti-cancer agents), or where the presence of specific pathophysiological processes is essential (eg anti-asthma drugs). Phase I studies are designed to investigate a new drug's pharmacokinetics, safety and, if practicable, its pharmacodynamics.

A1.3 The Declaration of Helsinki has articles that refer to non-therapeutic research and are appropriate to Phase I drug trials with certain exceptions.[1]

A1.4 In **Phase II studies** early therapeutic trials are undertaken, usually in a small number of closely monitored patients, to obtain information on efficacy, safety and their relationship with dose.

A1.5 **Phase III trials** are performed only when a drug is thought to have a reasonable probability of clinical usefulness and a good initial safety profile. These are the trials most commonly put before LRECs. They are designed to demonstrate whether or not a drug is effective for a particular clinical indication and to provide close monitoring of possible adverse effects in short and longer term trials. Phase III studies are usually randomised controlled trials. Uncontrolled ('open') studies are only seldom justified at this stage.

A1.6 **Phase IV studies** are carried out on licensed drugs and may be used to compare safety and efficacy with other established treatments and to investigate the effects of long term administration and adverse reactions. Trials to establish the efficacy of a licensed drug for a new clinical indication must undergo pre-registration trials; those are usually Phase III trials.

Official regulatory status

A1.7 An investigator should state the *exact regulatory status* of any drug to be used in the study and the committee should be told whether or not the intended trial is in accordance with the proposals assented to by the licensing authority (MCA). A study that departs from the provisions of the relevant certificate is unlawful.

1 CIOMS and WHO (1993), page 52

Product licences and certificates

A1.8 Product licences allow a drug to be marketed and define its indications. Trials with licensed drugs, but for 'new' indications (ie those not covered by the licence), require a Clinical Trial Certificate or Exemption (see below).

A1.9 Clinical Trial Certificates (CTCs) permit the use of unlicensed drugs, or of licensed drugs for 'new' indications. Manufacturers may, however, obtain an exemption from the need to hold a full CTC and may be granted a Clinical Trials Exemption Certificate (CTX) by the Medicines Control Agency (MCA). Most drug development in the UK is conducted under the CTX scheme.

A1.10 Doctors and dentists may obtain, from the MCA, an exemption (DDX) from the requirement to hold a CTC.

A1.11 Advice on regulatory matters and forms of application for CTX or DDX can be obtained from: *The Medicines Control Agency, Market Towers, Nine Elms Lane, Vauxhall, London, SW8 5NQ (telephone: 0171 273 3000).*

Exemption from the Medicines Act

A1.13 The Medicines Act provides exemption from licensing requirements if an unlicensed medicine is required to treat a particular (named) patient ('the named patient exemption'). It is not permissible to use this exemption to conduct research.

Licensing and ethics

A1.14 Issue of a certificate, licence or exemption by the MCA should not be used in a way that might cause patients or others to think that the study *ought* to be done or is guaranteed to be safe.

Duties of RECs

A1.15 The fact that a drug has been accorded a CTC, CTX or DDX does not imply that the ethics of the investigation have been subject to review, and in no way reduces the duties of RECs. There remains an obligation on investigators to satisfy themselves that they have the information necessary to make a judgement on the safety of the project they propose to undertake, and to satisfy the REC of this. If the committee rejects an application for a study under a CTX or DDX then the sponsor has a legal duty to inform the MCA forthwith.

A1.16 The grant of a CTC or CTX means that there has been some review or certification of the safety testing and quality of the product. The grant of a DDX does not necessarily involve any such review, and more responsibility, therefore, devolves upon the REC.

Healthy volunteers

A1.17 Studies involving healthy volunteers in the development of new drugs are outside the UK drug regulatory system and are not therefore covered by the CTC, CTX or DDX system. A particular obligation is therefore placed on LRECs to safeguard the well-being of participants.

A1.18 The reader is referred to the RCP document *Research on Healthy Volunteers* [1] and the ABPI *Guidelines for medical experiments in non-patient human volunteers*.[2].

Medicines Commission advice

A1.19 The Medicines Commission has been concerned about drug development studies in healthy volunteers. In 1987 it gave advice to the health ministers and this has been published. Selected quotations follow:

'Ethics committees should make it clear, if it is not already clear, that they

- require from applicants a certified statement that pre clinical investigations from which data have been submitted for their consideration have been carried out to a standard of no less than that required by the Department of Health under the clinical trial exemption (CTX) scheme; and in particular, because of the relevance to safety, that the quality and stability of the substance to be administered is assured;
- require, in submissions involving complex data, a succinct statement and/or an expert summary;
- seek outside expert opinion if necessary (for example because there was no member of the ethics committee who could guide the committee on the particular field of medicine to be covered in the healthy volunteer study);
- refuse applications which make inadequate provision for compensation for injury due to participation.'

'No healthy volunteer should be recruited for participation in a study without valid consent having been obtained beforehand. No approach should be made to those incapable of giving such valid consent such as mentally handicapped people, nor to people detained under the Mental Health Act, nor to prisoners, nor to people under the age of 18.'

'Every healthy volunteer should be informed of any consequence for employment or (personal) insurance status which may result from participation in a study.'

Pharmacovigilance/postmarketing surveillance

A1.20 Pharmacovigilance is concerned with assessing the safety of licensed medicines. These studies may be organised by pharmaceutical companies to collect data, primarily on safety, on their own products as used in everyday clinical practice and in accordance with the company's data sheet. Guidelines for the safety assessment of marketed medicines (SAMM) studies have been agreed between the ABPI, the BMA, the Committee on Safety of Medicines, the MCA and the Royal College of General

1 Royal College of Physicians (1986a)

2 ABPI (1990)

Practitioners.[1] The guidelines provide that plans of all such studies conducted by pharmaceutical companies should be filed in a register held by the MCA. ABPI have published guidelines for Phase IV clinical trials.[2]

Pharmacovigilance studies which are purely observational and unintrusive, and are concerned with collecting data *after* a decision to prescribe a particular product has been made, do not require approval from an LREC. Other forms of pharmacovigilance may do so.

1 ABPI, BMA, CSM, Royal College of General Practitioners (1988)

2 ABPI (1993a)

APPENDIX B

Use of medical records, registers or existing biological samples in research: the need for ethical review

A working party, with a strong lay membership concluded that to require formal ethical review of research involving personal medical records or stored biological samples alone is likely to delay or even inhibit valuable research: they further recommended, provided that such research is carried out with scrupulous confidentiality, it is by its nature harmless and does not require submission to an LREC. After careful consideration, Council of the RCP agreed to publish this report which is summarised below and has been published in full.[1]

Research involving access to medical records, registers, or existing biological samples only, without direct patient contact or involvement, is not considered to require individual patient consent or independent ethical approval provided that:

- explicit consent to access a patient's records is obtained either from the official custodian of those records or from the patient's clinician: the decision to access personal medical information should not be left to the sole discretion of the investigator;
- confidentiality is assured through adherence to professional ethical codes of conduct;
- the recipient of the information is a senior professional person eg a consultant medical practitioner or a principal in general practice who is subject to an effective disciplinary code enforced by his or her professional body over any breach of confidentiality, eg by suspension from practice in a serious case.

All research involving *direct contact* with patients or healthy subjects requires individual consent and independent ethical review.

1 Royal College of Physicians (1994)

APPENDIX C

Abbreviations

ABPI	Association of the British Pharmaceutical Industry
BMA	British Medical Association
BPA	British Paediatric Association
CIOMS	Council for International Organisations of Medical Sciences
CTC	Clinical Trial Certificate
CTX	Clinical Trial Exemption
DDX	Doctor's and Dentist's exemption
DHC	District Health Commission
DoH	Department of Health
EU	European Union
FDA	Food and Drug Administration
GMC	General Medical Council
GTAC	Gene Therapy Advisory Committee
HA	Health Authority
HIV/AIDS	Human Immuno Deficiency Virus/Acquired Immune Deficiency Syndrome
HFEA	Human Fertilisation and Embryology Authority
LREC	Local Research Ethics Committee
MCA	Medicines Control Agency
MRC	Medical Research Council
MREC	Multi-location Research Ethics Committee
NHS	National Health Service
NIH	National Institutes of Health
PIS	Patient (or subject) Information Sheet
RCP	Royal College of Physicians (of London)
RHA	Regional Health Authority
SAMM	Safety Assessment of Marketed Medicines
WHO	World Health Organisation
WMA	World Medical Association

REFERENCES

ABPI, BMA, CSM and Royal College of General Practitioners (1988). Guidelines on post-marketing surveillance. *Br Med J*;**296**:399–400. Also *Guidelines for company-sponsored safety assessment of marketed medicines* (SAMM Guidelines). London: MCA, Department of Health, 1993.

ABPI (1988). *Relationships between the medical profession and the pharmaceutical industry*. London: ABPI.

ABPI (1990). (1988, revised 1990). *Guidelines for medical experiments in non-patient human volunteers*. London: ABPI.

ABPI (1991). *Clinical trial compensation guidelines*. London: ABPI.

ABPI (1992). *Good clinical (research) practice*. London: ABPI.

ABPI (1993a). *Guidelines for Phase IV clinical trials*. London: ABPI.

ABPI (1993b). *Guidelines on the conduct of investigator site audits*. London: ABPI.

ABPI (1994). *Guidelines for ethical approval of human pharmacology studies carried out by pharmaceutical companies*. London: ABPI.

Bendall C (1994). *Standard operating procedures for Local Research Ethics Committees: comments and examples*. London: McKenna and Company.

Bendall C and Riddell J (1994). *Using standards for Local Research Ethics Committees: a guide to using the framework of standards and the standard operating procedures*. Bristol: NHS Training Divison.

Bennett J C (1993). Inclusion of women in clinical trials: policies for population subgroups. Synopsis of a White Paper written by the Board on Health Sciences Policy of Institute of Medicine. *N Engl J Med*;**329**:288–92.

British Paediatric Association (1992). *Guidelines for the ethical conduct of medical research involving children*. London: British Paediatric Association.

British Paediatric Association and Royal College of Obstetricians and Gynaecologists (1991). *A checklist of questions to ask when evaluating research during pregnancy and following birth*. Report of a joint working party. London: British Paediatric Association and Royal College of Obstetricians and Gynaecologists.

British Psychological Society (1990). Ethical principles for conducting research with human participants. *The Psychologist*; June 1990:270–2.

Chalmers I and Chalmers T C (1990). Research Ethics Committees. *Br Med J*;**300**:395.

CIOMS and WHO (1991). *International guidelines for ethical review of epidemiological studies*. Geneva: WHO.

CIOMS and WHO (1993). *International ethical guidelines for biomedical research involving human subjects*. Geneva: WHO.

Department of Health (1991). *Local Research Ethics Committees* OHSG(91)5. London: Department of Health.

Department of Health (1995). *Guidance on the use of fetal tissue for research diagnosis and therapy*. London: Department of Health.

Dudley H A F (1994). Research ethics committees and military defence. *J R Coll Physicians Lond*;**28**: 237–241.

EC (1990). *Notes for guidance on good clinical practice for trials on medicinal products in the European Community*. (Committee on Proprietary Medicinal Products) III/3976/88–EN.

EC (1991). *Updated standards for the testing of medicines for human use.* 91/507/EEC.

EC (1993). *The medical devices directive.* 1993/42 EEC.

Foster C G (1993). *Manual for Research Ethics Committees.* London: Centre of Medical Law and Ethics, Kings College.

Gene Therapy Advisory Committee (1994). *Guidance on making proposals to conduct gene therapy research.* London: Department of Health.

GMC (1987). *Professional conduct and discipline: fitness to practice.* London: GMC.

GMC (1995). Filming patients for television programmes. *News Review*;**7**:2.

Hall A S (1994). Context of consent. [Correspondence]. *Lancet*;**344**:618.

Irwig L, Glasziou P and March L (1995). Ethics of n-of-1 trials. [Correspondence]. *Lancet*;**345**:469.

King's Fund (1994). *Hospital accreditation programme: organisational standards and criteria.* (3rd edn). London: King's Fund.

Lancet Editorial (1992). Zelen protocols. *Lancet*;**339**:1574–5.

Law Commission (1995). *Mental incapacity.* (Law Commission No 231). London: HMSO.

Leigh and Barron Consulting Limited and Christie Associates (1994). *Standards for Local Research Ethics Committees: a framework for ethical review.* London: Department of Health.

McPherson K (1974). Statistics: The problem of examining accumulating data more than once. *N Engl J Med*;**290**:501–2.

Merkatz R B, Temple R, Sobel S, Feiden K and Kessler DA (1993). Women in clinical trials of new drugs. A change in Food and Drug Administration policy. Report of a working group. *N Engl J Med*;**329**:292–6.

Merck manual of diagnosis and therapy (1992). (16th edn). USA: Merck, Sharp and Dhome.

MRC (1985). *Responsibility in the use of personal medical information for research: principles and guide to practice.* London: MRC.

MRC (1991a). *Responsibility in investigations on human participants and material and on personal information.* London: MRC.

MRC (1991b). *The ethical conduct of research on children.* London: MRC.

MRC (1991c). *The ethical conduct of research on the mentally incapacitated.* London: MRC.

MRC (1991d). *The ethical conduct of AIDS vaccine trials.* London: MRC.

MRC (1994). *The health of the UK's elderly people.* London: MRC.

Moore v Regents of the University of California. See Appendix to *Human tissues: ethical and legal issues.* Report of the Nuffield Council on Bioethics, 1995.

Neuberger J (1992). *Ethics and health care.* King's Fund Institute Research Report. London: King's Fund.

Nicholson R H (1986). *Medical research with children: ethics, law and practice.* Oxford: Oxford University Press.

Nuffield Council on Bioethics (1995). *Human tissues: ethical and legal issues.* London: Nuffield Council on Bioethics.

Polkinghorne (1989). *Review of the guidance on the research use of fetuses and fetal material.* (Polkinghorne Report). Presented to Parliament, Cm 762. London: HMSO.

Royal College of General Practitioners (1993). *The importance of ethical considerations. Statement on the use of video recording of general practice consultations for teaching, learning and assessment.* London: Royal College of General Practitioners.

Royal College of Psychiatrists (1989). *Guidelines for ethics of research committees on psychiatric research involving human subjects*. Report of a working party. London: Royal College of Psychiatrists.

Royal College of Physicians (1986a) *Research on healthy volunteers*. Report of a working party. London: Royal College of Physicians.

Royal College of Physicians (1986b). *The relationship between physicians and the pharmaceutical industry*. Report of a working party. London: Royal College of Physicians.

Royal College of Physicians (1990). *Research involving patients*. Report of a working party. London: Royal College of Physicians.

Royal College of Physicians (1991). *Fraud and misconduct in medical research: Causes, investigation and prevention*. Report of a working party. London: Royal College of Physicians.

Royal College of Physicians (1994). Independant ethical review of studies involving personal medical records. Report of a working group. *J Roy Coll Physicians Lond*;**28**:429–43.

Silverman W A (1994). Patients preferences and randomised trials. *Lancet;* **343**: 1586.

Tobias J S and Souhami R L (1993). Fully informed consent can be needlessly cruel. *Br Med Journal*; **307**:1199–201.

West Berkshire Health Authority (1989). *Mental Health Act Commission intervening*. House of Lords 1989 2 A11 E.R.545.

World Medical Association Declaration of Helsinki (1989). (1964, revised 1989). *The World Medical Association Handbook of Declarations*.

Bibliography not directly referenced, quoted in the previous edition and considered useful

Department of Health, Education and Welfare (1979). *Protection of human subjects* (Belmont Report). Washington, USA: Department of Health, Education and Welfare.

Faculty of Occupational Medicine (1993). *Guidance on ethics for occupational physicians*. (4th edition). London: Royal College of Physicians.

Medical Research Council of Canada (1987). *Towards an international ethic for research with human beings*. Proceedings of the International Summit Conference on Bioethics April 1987, Ottawa.

INDEX

Bold type indicates pages on which subjects are discussed in depth

Notes

Notes

Notes